SELF-ASSESSMENT IN
OBSTETRICS & GYNAECOLOGY

SELF-ASSESSMENT IN
OBSTETRICS &
GYNAECOLOGY

JOHN STUDD

MD, MRCOG
Consultant Obstetrician and Gynaecologist,
King's College Hospital, London

DONALD GIBB

BSc, MRCP, MRCOG
Lecturer in Obstetrics and Gynaecology,
National University of Singapore, Singapore

IAN BROWN

FRCOG
Professor of Obstetrics and Gynaecology,
University of Zimbabwe, Zimbabwe

BLACKWELL SCIENTIFIC PUBLICATIONS

OXFORD LONDON EDINBURGH

BOSTON MELBOURNE

© 1983 by
Blackwell Scientific Publications
Editorial offices:
Osney Mead, Oxford, OX2 0EL
8 John Street, London, WC1N 2ES
9 Forrest Road, Edinburgh, EH1 2QH
52 Beacon Street, Boston
Massachusetts 02108, USA
99 Barry Street, Carlton
Victoria 3053, Australia

First published 1983

Photoset by Enset Ltd
Midsomer Norton, Bath, Avon
and printed and bound in
Great Britain by
Billings & Sons Ltd, Worcester

DISTRIBUTORS

USA
Blackwell Mosby Book Distributors
11830 Westline Industrial Drive
St Louis, Missouri 63141

Canada
Blackwell Mosby Book Distributors
120 Melford Drive, Scarborough
Ontario, M1B 2X4

Australia
Blackwell Scientific Book Distributors
31 Advantage Road, Highett
Victoria 3190

British Library
Cataloguing in Publication Data

Studd, John W.W.
Self-assessment in obstetrics &
gynaecology.
1. Gynecology—Examinations, questions, etc.
2. Obstetrics—Examinations, questions,
etc.
I. Title   II. Gibb, D.M.F.
III. Brown, Ian
618′.076   RG111

ISBN 0-632-01047-9

CONTENTS

PREFACE

This book is intended primarily for students preparing for examinations who may feel overwhelmed by the amount of work facing them and find themselves unable to plan their studies and subsequent revision. Self-assessment of existing knowledge and recognition of areas for further study is very important. This saves time being wasted on material with which the student is already familiar. Answering multiple choice questions is a method of self-assessment which is not time consuming, is thought provoking and can be fun.

Multiple choice questions have become firmly established in examinations and this should be considered a positive development from the student's point of view. Instead of essay questions on a narrow range of topics with which the student may not be familiar, an opportunity is presented to display a wider knowledge of the general subject. Greater objectivity and fairness and the availability of sophisticated computer technology to facilitate consistent and rapid marking have also stimulated the wider application of such questions.

In view of the differing formats of questions used in different centres these examples have not been produced as a trial run for an examination. They have been constructed to elaborate what we think are important teaching points at undergraduate level. The short comment after each answer is essential to the purpose of the book. Some answers may be debatable but in general the answers are consistent with the teaching of standard undergraduate texts. Controversy over answers is less evident at undergraduate level, than at postgraduate level but this in itself serves the purpose of stimulating further reading and critical thinking. The points discussed may appear as discussion subjects in viva examinations.

This book is not intended as a first reader for the undergraduate and it assumes basic reading of one of the standard undergraduate texts. It is not a short cut to passing examinations, but we hope it may improve studying efficiency. We emphasize that the format used in this book may not be that used in an examination; students should enquire about this from the relevant authorities at the medical school.

London 1983   *J.W.W.S.*
                                                                D.M.F.G.
                                                                    I.B.

THE MULTIPLE CHOICE QUESTION

FORMAT OF QUESTIONS

Several formats of multiple choice questions have been used. The most popular type in undergraduate examinations in the U.K. is the 'one best response' type. This begins with a stem followed by five possible completions. The candidate is asked to choose the best completions. Only one answer is acceptable but it is clear that there may be differing degrees of 'truth' in the other answers. One response is therefore considered *most* appropriate. In general this type of questions assesses the candidate's knowledge about one condition. An example is given below.

Example 1

The following are characteristic of primary syphilis:
A   an incubation period of 7 days
B   a painless ulcer
C   systemic upset
D   positive serology
E   all of the above

Only (B) is true but the other completions are also relevant to understanding the syphilitic process. The offered completions may include 'all of the above' or 'none of the above' which may be helpful to the candidate who only partially knows the answer.

Another common format is the 'multiple true/false' format which tests more knowledge, five points in each question, and is commonly used in postgraduate examinations. We have used this format as the most appropriate to the purpose of this book. The answers are usually clear but the ability to answer will depend on how much has been read about the subject. The following is an example.

Example 2

Ulceration of the vulva occurs in the following conditions:
A   gonorrhoea
B   chancroid

1

C   syphilis
D   candidiasis
E   Behcet's syndrome

Most students will know about gonorrhoea and candidiasis which are not associated with genital ulceration. They should also know about syphilis, but their knowledge of chancroid and Behcet's syndrome may be less certain. These diseases are linked as genital diseases but five different facts are tested.

Other types of questions exist such as the association of five entities correctly, choosing which item of a list is not associated with the stem, or more complex systems requiring skill in mental gymnastics. These are not popular in the U.K. as they cause as much confusion to the examiners as to the candidates and obscure the facts to be tested.

It is unlikely that more than one type will be included in an examination and the common type at undergraduate level is 'one best response'.

TERMINOLOGY

Terminological conventions are important and words like 'characteristic', 'associated', 'typical' and 'recognized' must be interpreted literally. Each word should be carefully considered but problems should not be sought by excessive analysis which the examiner clearly did not consider. Esoteric knowledge is not relevant and the answer will depend on well-established wisdom found in recent texts. This should not be taken to mean that clearly established modern advances are excluded. A statement that something occurs in a certain disease does not mean that it occurs all the time or that it occurs rarely, but that it occurs often enough to be associated with it. Numbers must be scrutinized and the denominator is of as much importance as the numerator given in a rate. Words that look or sound similar may be used to mislead the candidate who has not read the question carefully. Simple tricks may be built into the question but more elaborate deceptions are unlikely.

EXAMINATION TECHNIQUE

A logical and clearly defined approach to the examination is beneficial. The instructions must be carefully read and followed precisely.

It is important to know whether wrong answers lose marks or not. If so, guessing answers is likely to lose marks, whereas if marks are not lost then all questions should be answered even if it involves guessing. The candidate should find out from the medical school before the examination as it is likely that wrong answers will be penalized even at undergraduate level.

Read the question with each alternative completion. It should make grammatical sense. When an answer is selected mark it initially on the question sheet. Read it again looking for catches and when satisfied mark the answer card.

The answer card may be a computer card which should be marked with great care in the correct direction. A computer does not forgive basic errors such as marking the boxes in the wrong sequence. Leaving all responses to be transferred to the answer card at the end of the examination is foolish as time may run out and although the questions are answered the computer receives nothing.

There may be a place for leaving answers about which the candidate is uncertain until the end of the examination especially if marks are deducted for wrong answers. In that case a decision about the need for an extra mark compared with the risk of losing one will have to be made. In undergraduate examinations this is generally not necessary and all questions should be answered.

GYNAECOLOGY

1 In the external genitalia
A the anterior and posterior wall of the empty vagina lie in apposition
B the urethra opens into the vestibule
C secretions arise from vaginal epithelial glands
D Bartholin's glands lie deep to the posterior ends of the labia majora
E the labia minora have hair follicles

2 The pH of the vagina
A is high during the reproductive years
B is dependent on epithelial glucogen
C falls after the menopause
D restricts the growth of pathogenic organisms
E is dependent on Doderlein's bacilli

3 The following statements about the lower part of the uterus are correct:
A The squamo-columnar junction is found at the internal os
B The uterine artery passes inferior to the ureter
C A parous cervix is slit-shaped
D Peritoneum covers the upper part of the vagina posteriorly
E The isthmus is part of the cervix

Gynaecological Answers

1 A True
B True
C False
D False
E False

The lumen of the empty vagina lies transversely; the blades of a speculum should not be inserted antero–posteriorly thereby traumatizing the sensitive urethral area. The urethra, Bartholin's glands and vagina open into the vestibule which is the area bounded by the clitoris, labia minora and fourchette. Bartholin's glands lie deep to the labia minora. The vagina itself does not produce glandular secretions. The labia minora are two sensitive folds of skin containing erectile tissue but devoid of hair follicles.

2 A False
B True
C False
D True
E True

The pH of the vagina is neutral or alkaline (high) before puberty and after the menopause. The acid pH of the reproductive years is maintained by the action of Doderlein's bacilli on vaginal epithelial glycogen. This acidic environment inhibits the spread of pathogens. Alterations in this flora, sometimes iatrogenic in origin, due to the administration of drugs especially antibiotics, may lead to vaginitis.

3 A False
B False
C True
D True
E False

On speculum examination observation may be made of the patient's parity and the squamo-columnar junction although not visible macro-scopically is located at the external os. Important facts for the surgeon are that the ureter passes inferior to the uterine artery 2 cm lateral to the cervix ('water flows under a bridge') and access may be gained to the peritoneal cavity by the upper posterior vagina and the Pouch of Douglas. The isthmus is that part of the uterus between the body and the cervix; it partly forms the lower segment during pregnancy and functionally is more closely related to the body of the uterus than to the cervix.

4 The Fallopian tube
  A possesses a cilial lining
  B is actively motile
  C is easily palpable on examination of the adnexae
  D is covered by peritoneum
  E has a thick muscle layer in the isthmus

5 The ovary
  A lies posterior to the broad ligament
  B receives its blood supply from a branch of the internal iliac artery
  C is covered by peritoneum
  D is sensitive to pressure
  E has lymphatic drainage to the para-aortic nodes

6 The following vessels are all branches of the internal iliac artery:
  A uterine artery
  B obliterated umbilical artery
  C pudendal artery
  D superior rectal artery
  E vaginal artery

4 A True
  B True
  C False
  D True
  E True

The Fallopian tube propels its contents towards the uterus by muscular action and by ciliary flow. Defects in this motility may lead to infertility or inappropriate implantation as in ectopic pregnancy. A normal Fallopian tube is not palpable on digital examination. Its covering of peritoneum means that pathology in the tube may lead to signs of peritonitis and the thick muscle coat of the isthmus with its narrow lumen is important in the natural history of ectopic pregnancy; there is less room for expansion of the gestation sac and a greater probability of tubal rupture.

5 A True
  B False
  C False
  D True
  E True

The position of the ovary varies but it usually lies near the pelvic side wall in an area bounded by the external iliac vein, the ureter and the internal iliac artery. Pelvic examination of the adnexae should be performed gently as the ovaries are very sensitive with extensive sensory nerve supply but they are devoid of peritoneum. The ovarian artery arises from the abdominal aorta below the origin of the renal arteries and the lymphatic drainage is therefore to this site.

6 A True
  B True
  C True
  D False
  E True

The genital tract except for the ovary receives its blood supply from branches of the anterior division of the internal iliac artery. Internal iliac artery ligation is an effective treatment in the management of intractable post-partum haemorrhage, although collateral vessels ensure that necrosis does not occur. In utero the umbilical artery is the terminal division of this artery.

7 **The lymphatic drainage from the uterine cervix is through the following lymph nodes:**
A   superficial femoral
B   superficial inguinal
C   external iliac
D   obturator
E   presacral

8 **The pudendal nerve carries the following nerves:**
A   sensory from the anterior part of the labia majora
B   sensory from the perineum
C   sensory from the lower part of the uterus
D   motor to the external anal sphincter
E   sensory from the clitoris

9 **The following structures support the uterus in postion:**
A   the broad ligament
B   the infundibulo-pelvic ligaments
C   the transverse cervical ligaments
D   the vagina
E   the transverse perineal muscles

10 **The urogenital diaphragm is pierced by the**
A   ureters
B   rectum
C   vagina
D   urethra
E   obturator nerve

7 A False
B False
C True
D True
E True

Knowledge of the lymphatic drainage of the pelvis is essential in the understanding of the spread of neoplasms. Vessels from the cervix pass laterally through the broad ligament or posteriorly through the utero-sacral ligaments. They drain to the internal, obturator and external iliac nodes but some pass directly to the common iliac nodes and pre-sacral nodes. Radical surgery for carcinoma must include removal of all these nodes.

8 A False
B True
C False
D True
E True

Block of the pudendal nerve only has limited effect on account of its various components. In particular the anterior structures of the external genitalia require additional local infiltration to achieve good analgesia. There is no effect on pain arising from the uterus and cervix. The external anal sphincter, levator and superficial perineal muscles all receive their motor supply from this nerve.

9 A False
B False
C True
D True
E False

The transverse cervical, pubo-cervical and utero-sacral ligaments (condensations of visceral pelvic fascia) provide the main supports of the uterus although the insertion of the levator ani muscles into the muscular vagina also provides some support. The broad ligament is not a true ligament, but a peritoneal fold containing loose connective tissue. During a 'repair' operation the most important part is the identification and apposition of the ligaments.

10 A False
B False
C True
D True
E False

The urogenital diaphragm or triangular ligament fills the space between the descending pubic rami. It consists of pelvic fascia investing the deep transverse perineal muscles also called the compressor urethrae. It is pierced by the vagina and urethra and should not be confused with the pelvic diaphragm consisting of the levator ani and coccygei muscles.

11 The following associations of types of epithelium are correct:
A   ciliated and uterine body
B   stratified squamous and vagina
C   transitional and bladder
D   columnar and cervix
E   urethra and transitional

12 The ovarian ligaments
A   contain the ureters
B   contain the ovarian arteries
C   are attached laterally to the pelvic wall
D   lie anterior to the broad ligament
E   are homologous to part of the gubernaculum testis in the male

13 During the menstrual cycle
A   ovulation coincides with menstruation
B   the secretory phase of the cycle is of constant length
C   anovular cycles are characteristically painless
D   menstrual blood loss is 100 ml on average
E   libido is maximal at the time of ovulation

14 The luteal phase of the menstrual cycle is associated with
A   high luteinizing hormone levels
B   high progesterone levels
C   high prolactin levels
D   low basal body temperature
E   secretory changes in the endometrium

11 A False
  B True
  C True
  D True
  E True

The urinary tract is principally lined by transitional epithelium. The columnar epithelium of the cervix meets the stratified squamous of the vagina at the external os; the squamo-columnar junction. Contrary to popular belief the vagina does not have a mucous membrane as the squamous epithelium is devoid of glands: ciliated epithelial cells are confined to the Fallopian tube.

12 A False
  B False
  C False
  D False
  E True

The 'ligaments' of the pelvis are fibromuscular bundles of connective tissue. The ovarian ligament passes medially from the ovary to the uterus near the cornu posterior to the broad ligament, has no function in the adult but with the round ligament is homologous with the gubernaculum testis in the male.

13 A False
  B True
  C True
  D False
  E False

During the normal menstrual cycle ovulation occurs at mid-cycle and the second half (the luteal phase) remains constant irrespective of the overall length of the cycle. Anovular cycles are associated with less painful periods and hence the place of oral contraceptives in therapy. Unlike in the 'oestrus' of animals there is no association between ovulation and increased libido or sexual activity. Menstrual blood is between 40 and 80 ml.

14 A False
  B True
  C False
  D False
  E True

Follicle stimulating hormone (FSH) rises early in the cycle and at mid-cycle stimulating the granulosa cells of the follicle to secrete oestrogens. Luteinizing hormone (LH) rises to a sharp peak in mid-cycle precipitating ovulation which in turn is followed by development of the corpus luteum, elevated serum progesterone, a rise in body temperature and secretory changes in the endometrium. Prolactin levels are essentially unchanged during the menstrual cycle.

15 Fertilization

- **A** takes place in the uterine cavity
- **B** is accompanied by a surge of luteinizing hormone
- **C** is followed by extrusion of the first polar body
- **D** is facilitated by enzymes carried by the sperm
- **E** if effected by more than one sperm but only one ovum, will result in multiple pregnancy

16 The following are correct embryological associations:

- **A** germ cells and the wall of the yolk sac
- **B** Mullerian duct and female genital tract
- **C** Mullerian duct and Gartner's cyst
- **D** genital tubercle and clitoris
- **E** metanephros and kidney

15 A False
   B False
   C False
   D True
   E False

Ovulation is accompanied by a surge in luteinizing hormone and subsequent fertilization takes place in the distal end of the Fallopian tube. Hence ectopic pregnancy may result from failure of the ovum to proceed down the tube. Fertilization is followed by extrusion of the second polar body and subsequently the nuclei of ovum and sperm combine. Penetration of the zona pellucida of the ovum is dependent on hyaluronidase carried in the head of the sperm.

16 A True
   B True
   C False
   D True
   E True

The embryology of the genital tract is complex but is divided essentially into three parts: the development of the gonad, the internal duct system and the external genitalia. The ovary arises from mesodermal cells on the medial aspect of the uro-genital ridge (the genital ridge). All organs of the genito-urinary system except the bladder, urethra and vulva develop from the uro-genital ridge. However, germ cells themselves differentiate from the endoderm of the dorsal part of the hindgut (the wall of the yolk sac) and migrate through the root of the mesentery to reach the genital ridge. The female duct system arises from the Mullerian (M for mother) duct and the male duct system from the Wolffian duct. Every early embryo possesses both systems. Persistence and enlargement of the Wolffian duct in the female as Gartner's duct may manifest as a cyst. The genital tubercule becomes the penis or clitoris and the metanephros becomes the kidney.

17 In the process of germinal cell division
A   the ovary has its maximum number of cells at birth
B   the primary oocyte is haploid
C   the spermatozoon is haploid
D   the second reduction division in the male occurs after fertilization
E   diploid cells have forty-four autosomes

18 The following karyotypes are appropriate:
A   Turner's syndrome: 45XO
B   Testicular feminization: 46XY
C   Klinefelter's syndrome: 47XXY
D   Superfemale: 47XXX
E   Mongolism: 47 trisomy 21

19 The Barr body
A   arises from the Y chromosome
B   is found in Turner's syndrome
C   is found in Kinefelter's syndrome
D   is found near the cell membrane on microscopic examination
E   occurs in 10% of normal males

17 A False
B False
C True
D False
E True

The ovary has its maximum number of cells during the sixth month of intra-uterine development and at birth this number has already diminished. Most of the 2,000,000 oocytes present at birth are destined to be lost by atresia and only a few hundred will ovulate during the reproductive life span. Germ cells undergo reduction division (meiosis) resulting in the haploid ovum and spermatozoon but the primary oocyte is diploid. Normal diploid cells possess forty-four autosomes and two sex chromosomes. Meiosis is arrested during the first reduction division and this is not completed until after ovulation. The second reduction division occurs after fertilization in the female.

18 A True
B True
C True
D True
E True

Patients with Turner's syndrome are XO or mosaic having female external genitalia but being infertile due to gonadal dysgenesis. Those with testicular feminization are externally female although chromosomally male. They produce normal quantities of male sex hormones, but the developing external genitalia are resistant to the masculinizing effect. Patients with Klinefelter's syndrome are externally male but are infertile. Females with XXX complement are normal fertile females except for an increased incidence of mental retardation.

19 A False
B False
C True
D False
E False

The Barr body is the product of every X chromosome in excess of one. It therefore does not occur in males or Turner's syndrome but is found in males who have more than one X chromosome such as those with Klinefelter's syndrome. It lies close to the nuclear plasma membrane and is visible using suitable staining techniques as a dark dot 2 μm in diameter. The investigation is important as 1 in 300 live-born children have an X chromosome abnormality. Neonates with ambiguous external genitalia should be investigated.

20 Ambiguous external genitalia at birth
A   are commonly due to congenital adrenal hyperplasia
B   are associated with drug ingestion during pregnancy
C   occur in testicular feminization syndrome
D   occur in true hermaphroditism
E   are commonly associated with an abnormal karyotype

21 Patients with testicular feminization syndrome
A   have well formed breasts
B   complain of secondary amenorrhoea
C   lack pubic hair
D   have XY karyotype
E   are liable to develop malignant change in the gonads

22 Transexual patients characteristically
A   have normal external genitalia
B   have abnormal karyotype
C   have abnormal hormone profiles
D   are of subnormal intelligence
E   are maladjusted socially

20 A True
   B True
   C False
   D True
   E False

The condition of ambiguous external genitalia at birth is most likely to be due to congenital adrenal hyperplasia or maternal ingestion of progestagenic steroids. The development of the external genitalia depends on the endocrine environment of the fetus. Those with the absence of certain adrenal enzymes (most commonly 21-hydroxylase) producing excessive amounts of androgens. A rare cause of ambiguous genitalia is true hermaphroditism. Testicular feminization usually presents later as primary amenorrhoea. A karyotype is an important investigation but is generally normal.

21 A True
   B False
   C True
   D True
   E True

This curious syndrome occurring in XY individuals appears to be due to an insensitivity of end-organs to circulating androgens present at a male level. Oestrogens are also present leading to normal breast formation and development of the external genitalia. They have no uterus being irreversibly amenorrhoeic and infertile. Malignant change is more likely in such gonads and they should be removed. Hormone replacement therapy is necessary.

22 A True
   B False
   C False
   D False
   E True

These unfortunate patients, who are often unhappy and maladjusted socially before treatment and sometimes after, have no detectable abnormality of anatomical, chromosomal or endocrine sex. They are often of normal or above normal intelligence. Departure from the sexual norm should be considered sympathetically and not stigmatized. Homosexuality is having a sexual propensity towards individuals of the same sex, transvestism is having the urge to adopt clothing and physical characteristics of the opposite sex and transexualism is the overwhelming desire to change sex by means of an operation. Transexuals should have full psychiatric assessment and only then surgery considered.

23 The following endoscopic techniques are appropriate to the conditions:

  A colposcopy and carcinoma of the endometrium
  B culdoscopy and sterilization
  C laparoscopy and in vitro fertilization
  D hysteroscopy and endometrial polyps
  E cystoscopy and staging of carcinoma of the cervix

24 Oestrogens

  A are synthesized from cholesterol
  B are secreted by the anterior pituitary gland
  C are secreted by the adrenal gland
  D are secreted by the stromal cells of the ovary
  E are principally excreted in the urine

23 A False
   B True
   C True
   D True
   E True

'Scopy', derived from the Greek verb 'to observe', is prefixed with the appropriate Greek-derived prefix for the part of the body involved. Colpos refers to the vagina; the cervix lies in the vaginal vault. Colposcopy is an important investigation in carcinoma of the cervix. The pelvic organs can be observed by an endoscope in the Pouch of Douglas and sterilization performed although this is infrequently performed today. Laparoscopy is used for infertility investigations and sterilization but more recently has been used for oocyte recovery as part of the in vitro fertilization procedure. Looking inside the uterine cavity (hysteroscopy) is less commonly used in clinical practice but is appropriate for manipulations within the uterine cavity. Examination under anaesthesia and cystoscopy is an important procedure in staging of carcinoma of the cervix.

24 A True
   B False
   C True
   D False
   E True

Sex steroid hormones are synthesized from the common precursor cholesterol. The granulosa and theca cells of the ovary, under the influence of pituitary stimulating hormones (FSH and LH), secrete oestrogens. However, the adrenal gland plays a minor role. During pregnancy the fetal adrenal gland produces Dihydro-epiandrosterone sulphate (DHAS) which is converted to oestrogen by the placenta, conjugated in the maternal liver and excreted as oestrone and oestriol in the urine. The placenta does not synthesize oestrogen 'de novo'.

25 Oestrogens cause

  A hypertrophy of the uterus
  B secretory endometrial changes
  C increased motility of the Fallopian tube
  D proliferation of vaginal epithelium
  E secretion of breast milk

26 Puberty

  A refers to the onset of menstruation
  B usually reaches completion before the age of 10 years
  C is associated with a growth spurt
  D is associated with anovular menstrual cycles
  E is associated with changes in body fat

27 The menopause

  A is synonymous with the climacteric
  B occurs on average at age 40 years
  C is characteristically associated with irregular vaginal bleeding
  D is associated with low oestrogen levels
  E is associated with high follicle-stimulating hormone levels

25 A True
B False
C True
D True
E False

The breast, uterus, Fallopian tubes, vagina and vulva are target organs for oestrogens. Oestrogens cause the enlargement of the uterus and proliferation of vaginal epithelium seen at puberty and in pregnancy; their withdrawal causes atrophy after the menopause. Proliferative endometrial changes in the first half of the menstrual cycle depend on oestrogens and the secretory changes of the second half on progesterone. Withdrawal of oestrogens causes endometrial shedding. Lactation depends on oestrogen to stimulate duct proliferation, progesterone to cause alveolar growth and prolactin and oxytocin to stimulate secretion.

26 A False
B False
C True
D True
E True

Puberty, including menarche (the onset of menstruation), is a sequence of events usually occurring between 11 and 14 years of age but dependent on heredity, nutrition and environment. Deposition of subcutaneous fat occurs, a growth spurt takes place and secondary sexual characteristics appear. The first few cycles are often anovular and painless.

27 A False
B False
C False
D True
E True

As the menarche is the onset of vaginal bleeding during puberty so the menopause is the cessation of vaginal bleeding during the climacteric. It occurs on average at age 50 years and may be associated with irregular vaginal bleeding in a minority of cases. This should be investigated as these patients are in the age group for genital tract malignancy. The low oestrogen levels due to ovarian failure cause the pituitary gland to be released from negative feedback and secrete large amounts of follicle-stimulating hormone (FSH).

28 Speculum examination in the non-pregnant patient may reveal
   A   Nabothian follicles
   B   cervical incompetence
   C   loss of the urethro-vesical angle
   D   carcinoma in situ
   E   cystocele

29 Cervical erosions
   A   are often asymptomatic
   B   show ulcerative features on microscopic examination
   C   are associated with pregnancy
   D   are associated with oral contraceptive use
   E   are associated with later development of cervical carcinoma

30 Cervical ectropion
   A   is frequently asymptomatic
   B   consists of squamous epithelium
   C   is related to trauma during childbirth
   D   is exaggerated by bi-valve speculum examination
   E   may be corrected by trachelorrhapy

28 A True
  B False
  C False
  D False
  E True

Vaginal speculum in the pregnant or non-pregnant patient commonly reveals retention cysts of the cervical glands; Nabothian cysts or follicles. Cervical incompetence may be suggested by the finding of an open os in patients with an appropriate history but only during pregnancy. Carcinoma in situ is a histological diagnosis and loss of the urethro-vesical angle a radiological one. Different types and degrees of prolapse may be seen on speculum examination.

29 A True
  B False
  C True
  D True
  E False

Cervical erosions, often asymptomatic, occur when the columnar epithelium of the cervical canal extends into the vaginal portion of the cervix. An erosion is not an ulcerating lesion nor is it infective. They are commonly associated with oral contraceptive use or pregnancy, suggesting an aetiology related to hormonal changes. If they are asymptomatic no treatment is required and there is no association with the later development of malignant disease.

30 A True
  B False
  C True
  D True
  E True

Cervical ectropion, a prolapse of cervical columnar epithelium, is frequently misdiagnosed as a cervical erosion. Like an erosion it is often asymptomatic and appears after damage to the cervix during childbirth. It is exaggerated by wide separation of the blades of a bi-valve speculum in the vaginal vault and if it is observed as the instrument is removed it is seen to recede. Definite symptoms or subsequent pregnancy wastage is an indication for trachelorrhapy.

31 In threatened abortion at 15 weeks gestation in a nulliparous patient
- **A** pain is characteristic
- **B** the internal os is often open
- **C** fainting is characteristic
- **D** an ultrasound scan can demonstrate viability
- **E** absence of fetal movements suggests non-viability

32 In ectopic pregnancy the following are characteristic:
- **A** less than 10 weeks amenorrhoea
- **B** abdominal pain occurring before vaginal bleeding
- **C** shoulder-tip pain
- **D** passage of decidual cast
- **E** negative pregnancy test

33 In hydatidiform mole the following are characteristic:
- **A** vaginal bleeding
- **B** inappropriate uterine size for the period of amenorrhoea
- **C** the passage of vesicles vaginally
- **D** snow-storm appearance on ultrasound examination
- **E** raised serum human placental lactogen levels (HPL)

31 A False
B False
C False
D True
E False

The difference between threatened and inevitable abortion is that in the latter pain is frequent and the cervical os opens with the presence of products of conception in the cervical canal. Fainting is associated with ectopic pregnancy. Primigravid patients do not feel fetal movements as early as 15 weeks and fetal viability can only be confirmed by progression of the pregnancy or ultrasound scan.

32 A True
B True
C True
D True
E False

Ectopic pregnancy characteristically presents before 10 weeks amenorrhoea with abdominal pain preceding vaginal bleeding. The abdominal pain is of peritoneal origin due to blood from the damaged tube irritating the peritoneum. This peritoneal irritation also causes nausea, vomiting, fainting and shoulder-tip pain. Only after the sac has become incompletely viable do the hormone levels drop and vaginal bleeding occurs due to withdrawal of oestrogens. Almost a diagnostic feature in ectopic pregnancy is passage of a decidual cast. The result of pregnancy is variable depending on the viability of the sac and hormone secretion.

33 A True
B True
C True
D True
E False

Hydatidiform mole presents with vaginal bleeding in almost all cases and the uterus is often inappropriate for dates (more frequently large than small). Passage of vesicles per vaginam is diagnostic as is a snow-storm appearance on ultrasound examination. The characteristic hormone marker in mole is raised levels of human gonadotrophin (HCG) which results in a positive pregnancy test even in dilution.

34 The following are associated with hydatidiform mole:

A thyrotoxicosis
B vomiting
C absence of fetal movement
D pre-eclamspsia
D ovarian cysts

35 Missed abortion

A occurs with blighted ovum
B presents with vomiting
C is diagnosed by X-ray
D is associated with coagulation defect
E is treated by evacuation of the uterus

36 Precocious puberty

A is constitutional in the majority of cases
B may initially manifest as precocious thelarche
C occurs with intra-cranial tumours
D occurs with ovarian tumours
E occurs in Albright's syndrome

34 A True
B True
C True
D True
E True

Amenorrhoea followed by irregular vaginal bleeding occurs in most cases of hydatidiform mole; thyrotoxicosis, excessive vomiting and a pre-eclamptic syndrome are also characteristic but only occur in a minority of cases. Absence of fetal movements is very likely except in the very rare cases of co-existent mole and live fetus probably arising from a twin pregnancy. Theca lutein cysts of the ovary occur, are hormone-dependent and resolve after evacuation of the mole.

35 A True
B False
C False
D True
E True

Missed abortion exists when a conception is non-viable in the absence of the classical signs of threatened abortion. It is the clinical condition associated with blighted ovum and characteristically presents with the history of the presence and subsequent absence of the symptoms of pregnancy during a period of amenorrhoea. The uterus is smaller than the dates suggest. If prolonged it is associated with coagulation defects. It is diagnosed clinically, confirmed by ultrasonic examination and treated by evacuation of the uterus.

36 A True
B True
C True
D True
E True

Precocious puberty, the onset of breast development (thelarche) before the age of 7 years or menstruation before 9 years, usually follows the sequence of normal puberty; breast development, growth spurt, pubic hair growth, menstruation and axillary hair growth. It is constitutional in the majority of cases with no underlying cause but more serious causes include intra-cranial tumours, previous encephalitis and oestrogen-secreting ovarian tumours. Albright's syndrome is polyostotic fibrous dysplasia, brown skin pigmentation and precocious puberty.

37 Ectopic pregnancy is reliably confirmed by
    A   ultrasound examination
    B   hysterosalpingogram
    C   laparoscopy
    D   pregnancy test
    E   hysteroscopy

38 Sequelae of ectopic pregnancy include
    A   fibroids
    B   recurrent ectopic pregnancy
    C   infertility
    D   abdominal pregnancy
    E   cervical incompetence

39 The following are consistent findings in ectopic pregnancy:
    A   shock
    B   temperature of 40°C
    C   vaginal discharge
    D   lower abdominal tenderness
    E   enlarged 'bulky' uterus

37 A False
  B False
  C True
  D False
  E False

Ectopic pregnancy is only reliably confirmed by direct inspection of the pelvic organs with a laparoscope. As it is a life-threatening condition other investigations waste valuable time, and admission to hospital for laparoscopy is mandatory if there is any suspicion. Pregnancy test may be positive or negative and even if positive does not distinguish intra-uterine from ectopic pregnancy: a common differential diagnosis. During ultrasonic examination it is uncommon to visualize a gestation sac and an empty uterine cavity; an essential obervation in these circumstances.

38 A False
  B True
  C True
  D True
  E False

It is the already damaged Fallopian tube which is susceptible to ectopic implantation of the conceptus and such tubes have an increased chance of this event recurring. With such damaged tubes there is also difficulty achieving an intra-uterine pregnancy. Abdominal pregnancy is probably almost always secondary to a tubal pregnancy freeing itself from its primary implantation site.

39 A False
  B False
  C False
  D True
  E True

The majority of ectopic pregnancies do not present with shock but are of the 'chronic' variety. The pathology is a slowly leaking gestation sac causing episodes of peritoneal irritation manifesting as abdominal pain. This gradual leak may be through the fimbrial end of the tube (tubal abortion). The hormonal secretion, as in intra-uterine pregnancy, causes hypertrophy and enlargement of the body of the uterus and decidualization of the endometrium. Acute pelvic inflammatory disease, a common differential diagnosis from ectopic may present with a temperature of 40°C, but the pregnancy temperature in ectopic is rarely above 38°C.

40 Spontaneous abortion is associated with
- **A** rubella
- **B** malformation of the zygote
- **C** malaria
- **D** incarceration of the retroverted gravid uterus
- **E** septate uterus

41 In spontaneous abortion
- **A** threatened abortion often becomes septic
- **B** complete abortion is commoner than incomplete abortion
- **C** inevitable abortion terminates as carneous mole
- **D** if bleeding is heavy oxytocin is given
- **E** sepsis is treated by antibiotics and subsequent evacuation

42 Vulval haematoma
- **A** follows normal delivery
- **B** causes pain
- **C** causes shock
- **D** is treated by packing
- **E** is treated conservatively

40 A True
B True
C True
D True
E True

Spontaneous abortion is common perhaps occurring in more than 20% of all pregnancies. The majority of these conceptions have abnormal chromosomal constitution. This is not likely to recur in subsequent pregnancies in which there is a high chance of success. Acute illnesses especially those associated with fever cause abortion but the fetus of the mother with rubella may survive and be born infected. Malformations of the uterus are associated with second trimester abortion. Retroversion is only a cause of abortion in the rare cases when the uterus is fixed, incarcerated and untreated.

41 A False
B False
C False
D False
E True

As the os is closed, threatened abortion does not become septic unless there has been some interference possibly to induce abortion. The incomplete variety is much commoner than the complete one especially in the first and early second trimester and if there is any doubt evacuation should be performed. Carneous mole is the result of missed abortion and the oxytocic drug required in abortion is ergometrine as the uterus in early pregnancy is less responsive to oxytocin. Septic products of conception should be removed surgically after an initial course of antibiotics.

42 A True
B True
C True
D False
E False

Vulval haematoma may result from a tear or an episiotomy being repaired with poor haemostasis but is also associated with a normal delivery. It is very painful and characteristically causes shock out of proportion to the blood loss. It must be treated definitively by incision, drainage, ligation of vessels, obliteration of the cavity, pressure and antibiotics.

43 The Abortion Act in the U.K.
A   was passed in 1967
B   cites three conditions under which termination may be performed
C   requires the signatures of two practitioners to agree to a case
D   requires notification to the Department of Health
E   states that abortion is available on demand

44 The following are associated with genital tract prolapse
A   ulceration
B   backache
C   dyspareunia
D   frequency of micturition
E   menstrual irregularity

45 Third degree uterine prolapse
A   is termed procidentia
B   involves inversion of the uterus
C   usually results from a deficient perineum
D   is characteristically associated with stress incontinence
E   is treated by abdominal hysterectomy

43 A True
    B False
    C True
    D True
    E False

Abortion in the U.K. is controlled by The Abortion Act of 1967. It does not approve abortion 'on demand' however interpretation of its four clauses is dependent on the attitude of the practitioners involved. Notification to the Department of Health is mandatory where a record is kept. Termination must be performed in approved hospital by a recognized specialist who may also be one of the signatories.

44 A True
    B True
    C False
    D True
    E False

Utero-vaginal prolapse causes local discomfort, backache, urinary and bowel symptoms. The backache is often positional being alleviated when the patient lies down. Frequency of micturition occurs when a cystocoele acts as a reservoir for residual urine which may become infected. Emptying of the residuum even without infection results in frequency. Although there may be some degree of mechanical problem during intercourse pain is not a common feature. Hormonal status is generally unchanged and menstruation unaffected.

45 A True
    B False
    C False
    D False
    E False

Third degree uterine prolapse occurs when the whole length of the vagina inverts but the uterus remains attached to the top of the vagina in its usual shape. It is easily palpable within the prolapse. A deficient perineum is a common occurrence in parous patients and has no direct relationship to prolapse as the main uterine supports are higher up. Prolapse and stress incontinence may occur together, but each commonly occurs without the other. Procidentia must be treated surgically by a vaginal approach in order to tighten the supporting ligament or recurrence will occur. Vaginal hysterectomy is the most appropriate procedure if fertility is not a consideration.

46 The following are associated with genital tract fistulae:
- **A** endometriosis
- **B** diverticular disease
- **C** carcinoma of the cervix
- **D** radiation
- **E** obstructed labour

47 Fistulae due to obstructed labour
- **A** are commonly uretero-vaginal
- **B** cause continuous urinary incontinence
- **C** are best repaired immediately after delivery
- **D** are usually repaired by an abdominal approach
- **E** are repaired by a sling operation.

48 Mobile retroversion of the uterus
- **A** is suspected when the cervix points anteriorly on speculum examination
- **B** occurs in 20% of women
- **C** is usually asymptomatic
- **D** occurs at 20 weeks gestation
- **E** occurs in the puerperium

46 A False
B True
C True
D True
E True

In the developing world the commonest genital tract fistulae are those due to prolonged obstructed labour, but in developed countries with more advanced medical services fistulae are more often a result of gynaecological surgery. Hysterectomy, extended hysterectomy and hysterectomy complicated by adhesions and distorted anatomy entail such a risk. Malignant disease and radiotherapy also cause fistulae. The peri-colic abscess of diverticular disease may rupture into the vagina and cause a colo-vaginal fistula.

47 A False
B True
C False
D False
E False

During prolonged obstructed labour the fetal head is compressed against the base of the bladder. The blood supply of the damaged area is compromised but the damaged area may not slough for several days. When it does so symptoms, principally constant urinary incontinence, occur. Such fistulae should not be repaired immediately although insertion of a urinary catheter and continuous bladder drainage may lead to closure of some small fistulae. After the tissues have recovered from the initial damage a vaginal approach to repair usually offers the best prospect of cure and this should be done by a specialist. Tissue grafting may be necessary. A sling operation is performed for stress incontinence.

48 A True
B True
C True
D False
E True

More than 20% of women have a retroverted uterus most of them symptomless especially if the uterus is mobile. Speculum examination reveals the cervix to be pointing forward in the vaginal vault and bimanual examination reveals the uterine body in the posterior fornix. Its size may be difficult to assess but its presence can be confirmed by rectal examination. The uterus rises out of the pelvis by 14 weeks gestation unless the uncommon complication of incarceration occurs. The involuting uterus may fall posteriorly in the puerperium.

49 Fixed retroversion of the uterus is associated with

- **A** dyspareunia
- **B** pelvic pain
- **C** infertility
- **D** fibroids
- **E** pelvic infection

50 Retroversion of the uterus may be corrected by

- **A** Gilliam's operation
- **B** a Hodge pessary
- **C** pelvic floor repair
- **D** a sling operation
- **E** a laparoscopic procedure

51 Monilial infection of the vulva is associated with

- **A** pregnancy
- **B** the presence of an intra-uterine contraceptive device
- **C** diabetes mellitus
- **D** systemic antibiotic therapy
- **E** Bartholonitis

52 A Bartholin's abscess

- **A** is commonly due to gonorrhoea
- **B** is treated by excision
- **C** is frequently bilateral
- **D** is painful
- **E** causes peri-urethral swelling

49 A True
   B True
   C True
   D False
   E True

Fixed retroversion of the uterus is associated with the symptoms of the underlying disease which is usually endometriosis or pelvic infection. These symptoms include dysmenorrhoea, deep dyspareunia, low backache and pelvic pain. These conditions also cause infertility and the treatment may include correction of the retroversion.

50 A True
   B True
   C False
   D False
   E True

Correction of uterine retroversion may be effected by use of a Hodge pessary, the upper part of which puts tension on the utero-sacral ligaments. If it is doubtful whether symptoms are related to retroversion then a pessary test may be performed; the patient is observed for several weeks after insertion and if symptoms are consistently relieved then the retroversion should be definitely treated. Surgical treatment is by open ventrosuspension (Gilliam's operation) or sometimes may be performed by manipulation and ventrosuspension using a laparoscope.

51 A True
   B False
   C True
   D True
   E False

Candidiasis, monilial infection, is associated with diabetes mellitus because the glucose in the urine encourages fungal growth. It is also associated with oral contraceptive use and pregnancy even in the absence of glycosuria. Systemic antibiotic therapy affects the flora of the genital tract and may allow relative pathogens to flourish. Bartholin's gland infection is not caused by monilia.

52 A False
   B False
   C False
   D True
   E False

Infection of the Bartholin's gland is most commonly due to *Escherichia coli* or *Staphylococcus* although *Neisseria gonorrhoea* may sometimes be involved. It is typically unilateral causing swelling at the posterior end of the labium minus and great pain. It is treated by bed rest, antibiotics and marsupialization. Attempted excision of an actively inflamed cyst is likely to be difficult and accompanied by much haemorrhage. A chronic cyst or infection may require definitive excision.

53 Tuberculosis of the genital tract
A is characteristically bovine in origin
B commonly involves the vagina
C causes infertility
D is frequently associated with an abormal chest radiograph
E occurs in virgins

54 Tuberculosis of the genital tract
A is diagnosed by culture of vaginal discharge
B is diagnosed by culture of endometrial curettings
C is treated surgically in the first instance
D when treated aggressively is associated with frequent return of fertility
E is associated with ectopic pregnancy

55 Acute pelvic infection is associated with
A first trimester of pregnancy
B spontaneous abortion
C syphilis
D appendicitis
E the menopause

53 A False
B False
C True
D False
E True

Tuberculosis of the genital tract is usually due to post-primary haematogenous spread of pulmonary disease of human origin. However, the chest X-ray is unlikely to show an active focus and may be normal. Tuberculosis affects the Fallopian tubes and endometrium most commonly and only rarely the cervix, vagina and vulva. It is a potent cause of infertility in endemic areas. Signs of pelvic inflammation in a virgin suggest tuberculosis as the cause.

54 A False
B True
C False
D False
E True

Tuberculosis, whilst it may be diagnosed on careful examination and culture of menstrual blood in an at risk case, will not be diagnosed on examination of vaginal discharge. Examination of uterine curettings histologically and after staining by Ziehl–Neelson's method may be rewarding but longer term culture or inoculation into guinea-pig may be necessary. It should be treated medically in the first instance but results in terms of return of normal tubal function and fertility are disappointing.

55 A False
B True
C False
D True
E False

Acute pelvic infection characteristically may occur after abortion or delivery and with gonorrhoeal infection. Inflammation of the intestinal tract may affect the pelvic organs especially the right Fallopian tube in appendicitis. Tuberculosis is the only infection which may arise from haematogenous spread. Although lower abdominal discomfort is common in the first trimester of pregnancy the co-existence of pregnancy and acute pelvic inflammation is unlikely. Episodes of infection occur during reproductive life and are rare after the menopause.

56 **Acute salpingo-oophoritis is caused by the following organisms:**
  A *Streptococcus faecalis*
  B *Chlamydia*
  C *Toxoplasma gondii*
  D *Trichomonas vaginalis*
  E *Schistosoma mansoni*

57 **The following are characteristic symptoms in acute pelvic inflammatory disease:**
  A amenorrhoea
  B short episodes of acute abdominal pain
  C unilateral abdominal pain
  D rigors
  E shoulder-tip pain

58 **The following tests may be frequently expected to aid in planning the antibiotic therapy in pelvic inflammatory disease:**
  A microscopy of vaginal discharge
  B culture of vaginal discharge
  C gonoccal complement fixation test
  D culture of contents of pyosalpinx
  E culture of tubal swab obtained at laparoscopy

56 A True
   B True
   C False
   D False
   E False

Acute pelvic inflammatory disease is most commonly due to *Staphylococcus* and *Streptococcus* although *Chlamydia* is becoming increasingly implicated. Culture is difficult and this is reflected in the apparently differing incidences from centre to centre. Toxoplasmosis is a systemic infection with serious effects in pregnancy whilst trichomoniasis is an infection of the lower genital tract. Schistosomiasis is associated with lesions of the vulva, vagina and cervix and Fallopian tube but does not cause acute salpingo-oophoritis.

57 A False
   B False
   C False
   D True
   E False

Acute pelvic inflammatory disease may be difficult to differentiate from ectopic pregnancy. Menorrhagia and congestive dysmenorrhoea are more likely than amenorrhoea in pelvic inflammation. Pain is persistent, bilateral and signs of generalized peritonitis may develop. Fever, rigors and anorexia are characteristic in severe cases. Shoulder-tip pain due to sub-diaphragmatic irritation is more commonly seen in ectopic pregnancy; it is due to the tracking of blood.

58 A False
   B False
   C False
   D False
   E True

Whilst it is an important microbiological principle to take swabs to guide antibiotic treatment it is not commonly of use with respect to pelvic inflammatory disease. The organisms causing inflammation in the tubes will rarely be found on examination or culture of vaginal specimens with the notable exception of carefully taken specimens for *Neisseria gonorrhoea*. The aspirate of a tubal mass is frequently sterile. Gonococcal Complement Fixation Test is non-specific. In centres where early laparoscopy is performed the diagnosis may be confirmed and indeed *Chlamydia* isolated from swabs taken from the end of the tube.

59 Ulceration of the vulva occurs in the following conditions:
A gonorrhoea
B chancroid
C syphilis
D candidiasis
E Behcet's syndrome

60 The following are characteristic of primary syphilis:
B an incubation period of 7 days
B a painless ulcer
C systemic upset
D positive serology
E a sore throat

61 The following are characteristic of secondary syphilis:
A a pruritic rash
B a chancre
C condylomata acuminata
D mouth lesions
E positive serology

62 The following tests are specific for syphilis:
A dark-ground illumination microscopy of vaginal discharge
B Wassermann reaction
C Frei test
D *Treponema pallidum* immobilization test (TPI)
E fluorescent treponemal antibody test (FTA)

59 A False
   B True
   C True
   D False
   E True

Ulceration of the vulva occurs with neoplastic and infective conditions. The primary chancre of syphilis develops as a painless ulcer most commonly on the vulva but sometimes on the vagina or cervix. The ulcer in chancroid (soft sore) is painful: this disease is caused by Ducrey's bacillus and inguinal adenitis is typical. Behcet's syndrome, a rare disease of unknown origin possibly auto-immune, manifests as ulcers on the vulva and oral cavity.

60 A False
   B True
   C False
   D False
   E False

The painless ulcer on the vulva, vagina or cervix may pass undetected occurring after an incubation period of more than 10 days. The local lymph nodes become enlarged and rubbery but do not usually suppurate. Serological testing does not become positive until 6 weeks after the appearance of the primary chancre.

61 A False
   B False
   C False
   D True
   E True

About 2 months after the appearance and subsequent disappearance of the chancre the signs of secondary syphilis appear. The maculo-papular rash predominantly on the trunk and limbs is non-irritating. Mouth lesion, 'mucous patches' may appear, as may a sore throat. *Condylomata acuminata* are viral in origin and differ from the flatter, grey-topped, moist *Condylomata lata* of syphilis. Serology is characteristically positive during this spreading phase of the disease.

62 A False
   B False
   C False
   D True
   E True

Syphilis is confirmed by the finding of treponemal organisms on the examination of serum exuded from the chancre by dark-ground illumination microscopy. The Wassermann reaction is non-specific and is positive in Yaws, common in the West Indian community. Serological confirmation is obtained from the TPI and FTA tests.

63 Chancroid

   A   is a viral condition
   B   presents as painful ulceration
   C   causes painful adenitis
   D   is associated with suppuration
   E   is treated with sulphonimades

64 The following symptoms are characteristically associated with uterine fibromyomata:

   A   dyspareunia
   B   dysmenorrhoea
   C   vaginal discharge
   D   abdominal pain
   E   menorrhagia

65 Fibromyomata

   A   are composed of striated muscle
   B   are very vascular
   C   have a true capsule
   D   frequently have calcium deposits
   E   occur in the uterine cervix

66 Uterine fibromyomata characteristically occur in:

   A   contraceptive pill users
   B   black patients
   C   smokers
   D   teenage girls
   E   infertile patients

63 A False
   B True
   C True
   D True
   E True

Chancroid is an infection caused by Ducrey's bacillus; an organism which is very difficult to isolate. Typically there is painful ulceration, sometimes multiple ulcers, on the vulva and vagina. There is associated lymph node enlargement which may procede to suppuration. It should be distinguished from syphilis. Pus should be aspirated and sulphonamides given. Resistant cases will need Streptomycin or tetracycline.

64 A False
   B False
   C False
   D False
   E True

Uterine fibromyomata, commonly called fibroids, are often symptomless although the patient may present with abdominal enlargement or menorrhagia. Dyspareunia, dysmenorrhoea, vaginal discharge and abdominal pain are unlikely unless there is a complication such as torsion haemorrhage, pelvic sepsis or endometriosis.

65 A False
   B False
   C False
   D False
   E True

Although myomectomy may be complicated by bleeding the fibromyoma itself is relatively avascular composed of smooth muscle and fibrous tissue surrounded by a false capsule of myometrium. Calcification is unusual, being found in a few tumours of long standing. Cervical fibromyomata occur.

66 A False
   B True
   C False
   D False
   E True

Uterine myomata occur in women who have never been pregnant or who have not been pregnant for some time. Once present they also cause infertility and abortion. They are more common in black patients. They are at least partially oestrogen dependent decreasing in size after the menopause but are not associated with contraceptive pill use.

67 The following changes in a fibromyoma cause symptoms:
A   hyaline degeneration
B   cystic degeneration
C   red degeneration
D   torsion
E   sarcomatous change

68 Red degeneration of a myoma characteristically:
A   occurs during pregnancy
B   causes pain
C   causes fever
D   is associated with a clotting defect
E   is treated surgically

69 Endometriosis characteristically occurs in women who are
A   in lower socio-economic group
B   perimenopausal
C   nulliparous
D   using IUCD
E   black

70 Characteristic symptoms of endometriosis include:
A   dysmenorrhoea
B   superficial dyspareunia
C   amenorrhoea
D   pre-menstrual tension
E   infertility

71 The following physical findings are consistent with a diagnosis of endometriosis:
A   fixed retroversion of the uterus
B   adnexal enlargement
C   nodules on rectal examination
D   vulval nodules
E   cervical lesions

67 A False
B False
C True
D True
E True

Hyaline degeneration, cystic degeneration and calcification of fibromyomata do not cause symptoms and are found on histological or radiological examination. Red degeneration, torsion and infection cause acute symptoms. Sarcomatous change which occurs in less than 0.2% of lesions may be suspected when there is pain and rapid increase in size especially after the menopause.

68 A True
B True
C True
D False
E False

Red degeneration of a myoma causing pain, tenderness and fever occurs during pregnancy and is due to obstruction of the venous drainage causing back pressure, rupture of vessels and extravasation of blood into the tumour. There is no associated clotting defect and treatment is conservative with pain relief and bed rest.

69 A False
B False
C True
D False
E False

Endometriosis is a disease of the higher socio-economic groups and is rare in black patients in Africa and the West Indies. It characteristically occurs in women who marry late but settles in the perimenopausal period disappearing after cyclical hormonal changes cease.

70 A True
B False
C False
D False
E True

25% of cases of endometriosis are asymptomatic; symptoms depend on the site of the lesions. Deep dyspareunia, dysmenorrhoea and menstrual irregularities; usually excessive or more frequent periods are common. Infertility may be the main complaint and is due to hormonal imbalance or defective tubal pick-up rather than tubal blockage.

71 A True
B True
C True
D True
E True

The commonest site of endometriosis is on the ovary and in the Pouch of Douglas. The utero-sacral ligaments may be thickened, the ovaries cystic and the recto-vaginal septum involved. The vulva may be involved and black endometriotic spots may appear on the cervix.

72 The following are effective in the treatment of endometriosis:
   A   clomiphene
   B   oophorectomy
   C   oral contraceptive
   D   danazol
   E   progestagens

73 Congenital abnormalities of the uterus are associated with:
   A   recurrent abortion
   B   hydatidiform mole
   C   amenorrhoea
   D   malpresentations
   E   abnormalities of the urinary tract

74 Primary amenorrhoea occurs in:
   A   testicular feminization syndrome
   B   oestrogen-secreting tumours
   C   intra-cranial tumours
   D   Turner's syndrome
   E   Down's syndrome

75 Secondary amenorrhoea occurs in:
   A   hyperprolactinaemia
   B   tuberculous endometritis
   C   Sheehan's syndrome
   D   anorexia nervosa
   E   polycystic ovarian syndrome

76 Menorrhagia is associated with:
   A   fibromyomata
   B   the menopause
   C   hypothyroidism
   D   chronic salpingo-oophoritis
   E   hyperprolactinaemia

72 **A** False   The aim of any hormone treatment is endometri-
   B True   osis to suppress cyclical hormone production. The
   C True   problem is that to achieve this aim, ovulation must
   D True   be suppressed in these infertile patients and side-
   E True   effects are common.

73 **A** True   Congenital malformation of the uterus may cause
   B False   recurrent abortion and pre-term labour. If there is
   C True   no endometrium connected with the vagina there
   D True   will be amenorrhoea. Mechanical problems may
   E True   occur in the third trimester and during labour caus-
                   ing malpresentations. Radiological investigation of
                   the urinary tract should be performed.

74 **A** True   The complete absence of menstruation in a female
   B False   may be due to a structural defect of the genital tract
   C True   or a functional defect rendering that endometrium
   D True   incapable of menstruation. Congenital abnormal-
   E False   ities such as absent uterus or the potentially revers-
                   ible imperforate hymen should be sought. Defects
                   of the hypothalamo-pituitary-ovarian axis are more
                   difficult to detect and treat.

75 **A** True   Secondary amenorrhoea and oligomenorrhoea have
   B True   similar aetiologies and represent the same factors on
   C True   a different time scale. Local causes such as tuber-
   D True   culous endometritis and Asherman's syndrome
   E True   (amenorrhoea traumatica) are rare and hypo-
                   thalamo-pituitary-ovarian axis defects are com-
                   moner.

76 **A** True   Excessive loss during menstruation is most com-
   B False   monly functional in origin due to hormonal imbal-
   C True   ance. However, organic lesions such as fibro-
   D True   myomata, neoplasia and ovarian involvement in
   E False   pelvic infection should be excluded. Hypo-
                   thyroidism should not be forgotten and bleeding
                   disorders are rarely responsible.

77 Spasmodic dysmenorrhoea characteristically:
  A occurs in the first cycles after the menarche
  B occurs on the first day of menstruation.
  C radiates to the thighs
  D responds to oral contraceptive therapy
  E responds to prostaglandin synthetase inhibitor therapy

78 The following structures are endocrinologically active:
  A corpus albicans
  B trophoblast
  C amnion
  D endometrium
  E corpus luteum

79 The anterior lobe of the pituitary gland secretes:
  A gonadotrophin-releasing hormone
  B luteinizing hormone
  C oxytocin
  D human placental lactogen
  E prolactin

80 The following organs respond to oestrogens:
  A breasts
  B Fallopian tube
  C uterine body
  D vaginal epithelium
  E cervical glands

81 The following are precursors of oestradiol:
  A cholesterol
  B stilboestrol
  C arachidonic acid
  D dehydroepiandrosterone
  E testosterone

77 A False
   B True
   C True
   D True
   E True

Spasmodic dysmenorrhoea occurs in the absence of obvious pelvic disease in young patients. It occurs when the myometrium contracts and is associated with ovular cycles; response to suppression of ovulation is good. Recent studies have found increased levels of prostaglandin in the menstrual fluid; response to drugs which inhibit prostaglandin synthesis also occurs.

78 A False
   B True
   C False
   D False
   E True

The corpus luteum and trophoblast are important secretors of hormones in early pregnancy. The corpus albicans is the inactive scar of a previous corpus luteum. The endometrium is only an end organ responding to hormonal stimulation and the amnion is not a significant secretor of hormones.

79 A False
   B True
   C False
   D False
   E True

Gonadotrophin-releasing hormone secreted by the hypothalamus stimulates the pituitary to secrete follicle-stimulating hormone (FSH) and luteinizing hormone (LH). Prolactin is secreted by the anterior pituitary and oxytocin by the posterior pituitary.

80 A True
   B True
   C True
   D True
   E True

Oestrogen is responsible for the development of the genital tract and secondary sexual characteristics. Fallopian tube motility is increased by oestrogens. Oestrogen causes breast development but progesterone, prolactin and oxytocin are necessary for lactation. The cervical mucus secreted by cervical glands depends upon oestrogen levels.

81 A True
   B False
   C False
   D True
   E True

All sex steroids originate from the conversion of acetate moieties to cholesterol. The synthetic pathway is complex but involves progesterone, epiandrosterone, androstenedione and testosterone. Stilboestrol is a synthetic compound with oestrogenic activity but is not a steroid molecule. Arachidonic acid is the precursor of prostaglandins.

82 Dysfunctional uterine bleeding occurs in:
   A   the menopause
   B   hypothyroidism
   C   carcinoma of the cervix
   D   pelvic inflammatory disease
   E   ectopic pregnancy

83 The following drugs enhance fertility in the short term:
   A   human menopausal gonadotrophin (HMG)
   B   conjugated equine oestrogens
   C   bromocriptine
   D   danazol
   E   clomiphene citrate

84 The following are side-effects of bromocriptine:
   A   multiple pregnancy
   B   vaginal dryness
   C   postural hypotension
   D   congenital abnormality
   E   menstrual irregularity

85 Hyperprolactinaemia is associated with:
   A   the use of chlorpromazine
   B   galactorrhoea
   C   ovarian cysts
   D   pituitary tumours
   E   amenorrhoea

82 A True
B True
C False
D False
E False

Dysfunctional uterine bleeding is defined as irregular bleeding in the absence of tumour, infection or pregnancy. It is most often due to sex hormone imbalance although hypothyroidism or bleeding disorders should be considered.

83 A True
B False
C True
D False
E True

Human menopausal gonadotrophin (HMG), containing follicle-stimulating hormone (FSH) and luteinizing hormone (LH) available commercially as Pergonal, stimulates the ovary and induces ovulation in patients with hypothalamo-pituitary dysfunction. Bromocriptine is effective in lowering the serum prolactin which inhibits ovulation in hyperprolactinaemia. Clomiphene citrate stimulates ovulation and is the most commonly used fertility drug. Exogenous oestrogens will suppress ovulation as does danazol.

84 A False
B False
C True
D False
E False

Bromocriptine has few side-effects but should be started in low dosage, taken at night, in case postural hypotension occurs. It will regularize menstruation and restore oestrogen status improving vaginal dryness. Although a fertility drug, it is not associated with multiple pregnancy as it only restores the normal hormonal milieu. The drug should be stopped if conception occurs but few congenital abnormalities have been recorded.

85 A True
B True
C False
D True
E True

Hyperprolactinaemia causes infertility with amenorrhoea/oligomenorrhoea and galactorrhoea in some cases. Drugs, such as chlorpromzine, tricyclic anti-depressants and methydopa, are the commonest cause. Ovarian cysts are not associated but the most serious cause of hyperprolactinaemia is a tumour of the anterior pituitary gland which must always be excluded.

86 Lactation is associated with
    A   reduced fertility
    B   spurt release of oxytocin
    C   high oestrogen levels
    D   high prolactin levels
    E   uterine contractions

87 The advantages of breast feeding include:
    A   reduced cost
    B   an improved mother–child relationship
    C   sterility of infant's intestinal contents
    D   reduced allergic disorders in the child
    E   more rapid loss of maternal fat

88 Lactation is suppressed by:
    A   stilboestrol
    B   breast binding
    C   expression of breast milk
    D   bromocriptine
    E   human placental lactogen

89 The following steroids are produced by the ovary
    A   progestagens
    B   androgens
    C   glucocorticoids
    D   mineralocorticoids
    E   oestriol

86 A True
B True
C False
D True
E True

Lactation causes amenorrhoea and reduced fertility but the contraceptive effect should not be depended upon. The hormonal support of lactation basically depends on a breast primed by oestrogen, progesterone and human placental lactogen, stimulated by prolactin and then provoked to eject milk by suckling-stimulated reflex release of oxytocin which contracts the myoepithelial elements. Oxytocin also stimulates uterine contractions: the 'after-pains'.

87 A True
B True
C False
D True
E True

Breast feeding has undergone a renaissance as its many advantages have been publicized. One striking result of artificial feeding in developing countries is an increased incidence of gastro-intestinal infection which may be lethal. However, intestinal flora in infants is always present and the advantage of breast feeding is the absence of pathogens. Mothers also regain their 'figure' more quickly when they breast feed.

88 A True
B True
C False
D True
E False

Oestrogens, such as stilboestrol, have been previously used to suppress lactation but their association with thrombo-embolism has resulted in the discontinuation of this practice. Simple breast binding is effective and should be combined with analgesia. Expression and stimulation of the breast results in continued secretion. In patients with specific problems such as stillbirth or neonatal death the more expensive bromocriptine may be used.

89 A True
B True
C False
D False
E False

The oestrogens produced by the ovary are principally oestradiol and oestrone; oestriol is an excretion product. The theca cells secrete progestagens and the stromal cells are important producers of androstenedione, dehydroepiandrosterone and testosterone. The ovary does not possess the enzymes necessary to produce glucocorticoids and mineralocorticoids.

90 Tubal patency may be confirmed by:
- **A** gynaecography
- **B** hysteroscopy
- **C** laparoscopy and passage of dye
- **D** insufflation of CO_2
- **E** hysterosalpingography

91 The following association of instruments and procedures are appropriate:
- **A** Vabra's aspirator and endometrial biopsy
- **B** Bierer's curette and menstrual regulation
- **C** Ayre's spatula and cervical cytology assessment
- **D** Karman's catheter and termination of pregnancy
- **E** Cusco's speculum and vaginal hysterectomy

92 The following are procedures performed vaginally:
- **A** staging of carcinoma of the ovary
- **B** Marshall–Marchetti operation
- **C** Manchester operation
- **D** trachelorrhapy
- **E** salpingolysis

90 A False
B False
C True
D True
E True

Patency of the Fallopian tubes was formerly established by tubal insufflation tests. Although sometimes useful they were unreliable and more recent technological progress has led to the use of the laparoscope with passage of dye and X-ray imaging of a radio-opaque dye passed through the tubes (hysterosalpingogram). Examination of the uterine cavity with a hysteroscope will not yield information concerning tubal patency.

91 A True
B False
C True
D True
E False

Vabra curette and aspirator is a useful apparatus for endometrial biopsy and outpatient curettage. Early termination of pregnancy and menstrual regulation is performed using a small plastic curette. The Bierer is an inflexible metal device. Papanicolaou smears are performed on cells obtained using an Ayre's spatula. During termination of pregnancy uterine size is assessed bi-manually and the flexible Karman's catheter is appropriate. Vaginal hysterectomy necessitates an open speculum like an Auvard's or Sims'.

92 A False
B False
C True
D True
E False

Staging of carcinoma of the ovary is performed at laparotomy whereas the other gynaecological neoplasm are staged on vaginal examination. The Manchester operation and trachelorrhapy are operations involving the cervix. Marshall–Marchetti operation, colpocystopexy is performed abdominally. Any tubal operation is a very delicate procedure and is performed under full vision from above.

93 Incontinence of urine occurs in:
A cystitis
B post-operative period of Wertheim's hysterectomy
C multiple sclerosis
D detrusor instability
E ectopic ureter

94 The following are suggestive of genuine stress incontinence:
A constant wetness
B passage of large amount of urine
C dysuria
D prolapse
E haematuria

95 Incontinence of urine is investigated by:
A colposcopy
B cystoscopy
C intravenous urography
D cystometry
E urodynamic investigations

96 The following techniques are used in the assessment of ovulation:
A X-rays
B ultrasound
C assay of human chorionic gonadotrophin
D observation of cervical mucus
E assay of serum progesterone

93 A True
  B False
  C True
  D True
  E True

Detrusor instability, sometimes associated with cystitis, causes urge incontinence because the reflex contraction of the detrusor muscle in the bladder causes emptying at relatively low volumes. Urge incontinence should be distinguished from stress incontinence and overflow incontinence occurring in neurological conditions because treatment is essentially different. Genito-urinary fistula, ectopia vesicae and ectopic ureter cause constant wetness. After Wertheim's hysterectomy the denervated bladder fails to contract and retention of urine occurs.

94 A False
  B False
  C False
  D False
  E False

Genuine stress incontinence due to a positive pressure gradient between bladder and urethra during stress presents as the painless passage of small amounts of normal urine. Constant wetness suggests a fistula or other structural problem. Prolapse may be associated with any kind of incontinence and haematuria suggests other pathology.

95 A False
  B True
  C True
  D True
  E True

A thorough investigation of the urinary tract should be performed in urinary incontinence because effective treatment is dependent on this assessment. Urodynamic tests and video cyto-urethrography will give the most information. A critical area is the structural and functional integrity of the bladder neck (the internal sphincter).

96 A False
  B True
  C False
  D True
  E True

The only conclusive evidence of ovulation is pregnancy but signs of luteinization of the follicle suggest it has occurred. End-organ response to progesterone secretion by the luteinized follicle includes specific changes in the endometrium, cervical mucus and vaginal cytology. Recently, follicle formation and rupture has been monitored by ultrasound.

97 In vaginal atresia
- **A** secondary sexual development is abnormal
- **B** a normal uterus is commonly present
- **C** Frank's procedure may be used
- **D** karyotype should be performed
- **E** Sheare's operation may be used

98 Sexual dysfunction is associated with:
- **A** negative attitudes to sexuality during upbringing
- **B** previous sexual assault
- **C** masturbation during adolescence
- **D** recent childbirth
- **E** inexpert episiotomy repair

99 Clomiphene
- **A** directly stimulates ovulation
- **B** causes hot flushes
- **C** is associated with congenital malformation
- **D** is given for 21 days each cycle
- **E** causes follicle-stimulating hormone (FSH) to rise

97 A False
   B False
   C True
   D True
   E True

Absence of the vagina suggests abnormality or absence of Mullerian duct development. However, the ovaries being of different embryological origin develop normally and hormonal stimulus causes secondary sexual development. Karyotype should be performed to distinguish vaginal atresia from testicular feminization (XY karyotype). Various procedures have been used including pressure on the vulva by dilators as proposed by Franks. Williams' operation and McIndoe–Read procedure are used in U.K. and U.S.A. Sheare's operation, as used in Singapore, to locate and dilate the embryological remnant is physiological and successful.

98 A True
   B True
   C False
   D True
   E True

The patient with sexual problems should initially be assessed for structural abnormalities. A previous vaginal repair procedure done too tightly may cause dyspareunia. The commoner association with sexual dysfunction include faulty attitudes during upbringing, inadequate sex education and maladjustment. Women adjusting to their new role as mother may experience problems especially if they do not perceive this as their chosen role.

99 A False
   B True
   C False
   D False
   E True

Clomiphene, used to induce ovulation, acts indirectly by occupying oestrogen receptors in the hypothalamus. This causes the hypothalamus to perceive low endogenous oestrogen levels and so increase the pituitary output of follicle-stimulating hormone. It is given for 5 days each cycle, causes side-effects of vasomotor flushes, bloating, breast discomfort and visual symptoms. There is no increase in congenital malformation.

100 Human menopausal gonadotrophin (HMG) used to stimulate ovulation:
A   is given orally
B   necessitates monitoring of endogenous oestrogens
C   causes ovarian enlargement
D   causes multiple pregnancies
E   is used in conjunction with human chorionic gonadotrophin (HCG) injections

101 In male reproductive physiology
A   spermatogenesis is completed in about 35 days
B   luteinizing hormone stimulates the Leydig cells to produce testosterone
C   prolactin plays an important part
D   testicular temperature is important
E   frequent ejaculation affects the sperm count

102 The following are symptoms of the climacteric
A   obesity
B   pre-menstrual tension
C   formication
D   menorrhagia
E   headache

103 In anorexia nervosa in females
A   secondary amenorrhoea is a recognized feature
B   endogenous oestrogen levels are low
C   follicle-stimulating hormone (FSH) levels are high
D   lanugo hair occurs
E   marriage leads to improvement

100 A False
  B True
  C True
  D True
  E True

Gonadotrophin therapy for anovulation is expensive and associated with significant complications. A series of injections of HMG are followed by an injection of HCG when the ovaries show signs of follicular development. This is monitored by serum oestrogens or ultrasound. Multiple pregnancies occur as does the hyperstimulation syndrome.

101 A False
  B True
  C False
  D True
  E True

Spermatogenesis takes 90 days to complete. Follicle-stimulating hormone affects the process of spermatogenesis and luteinizing hormone stimulates testosterone secretion. Prolactin does not have a major role in spermatogenesis. The process is affected by temperature and tight underwear will raise the testicular temperature by holding the testes close to the body reducing fertility. Frequent ejaculation lowers the sperm count.

102 A False
  B False
  C True
  D False
  E True

The most characteristic features of the climacteric are the vasomotor symptoms of hot flushes, sweats and headaches. Menstrual disturbances are not regarded as a normal feature of the approaching menopause. The itching under the skin known as formication is unusual but characteristic.

103 A True
  B True
  C False
  D True
  E False

Anorexia nervosa is a psychological disorder with endocrine manifestations through hypothalamic mediation. FSH and LH levels are low with consequent low oestrogen levels and secondary amenorrhoea. There is a generalized reappearance of lanugo hair. It is more common in the higher social classes and marriage institutionalizes the disorder, perpetuating it.

104 Characteristic features of Klinefelter's syndrome include

A mental retardation
B oligospermia
C gynaecomastia
D XXY genotype
E congenital heart disease

105 In true hermaphroditism

A external sex is usually female
B chromosomal sex is usually female (46XX)
C mosaics do not occur
D primordial follicles and seminiferous tubules are both present
E end-organ resistance is a feature

106 The following features are visible in a fresh saline preparation of a vaginal discharge examined microscopically:

A epithelial cells
B *Neisseria gonorrhoea*
C *Trichomonas vaginalis*
D *Candida albicans* mycelia
E spermatozoa

107 The following features are characteristic of cervical mucus in mid-cycle:

A increased quantity
B increased cellularity
C absence of arborization
D increased viscosity
E the presence of red cells

108 Progestogen-only contraceptive pills

A are safer than combined pills for the patient over the age of 40 years
B produce amenorrhoea
C produce menorrhagia
D do not usually stop ovulation
E are taken every day of the month

104 A False
   B False
   C True
   D True
   E False

Klinefelter's syndrome occurs in phenotypic males with XXY genotype. Azoospermia is the rule and infertility a feature. Gynaecomastia and eunochoidism occur but congenital heart disease is not a feature. While patients with Klinefelter's syndrome are more often mentally retarded than other males, it is not a characteristic feature.

105 A False
   B True
   C False
   D True
   E False

In this condition both primordial follicles and seminiferous tubules are present in gonadal tissue. Chromosomal sex is usually 46XX. Mosaics do occur but external sex is predominantly male with a phallus while a uterus is commonly present.

106 A True
   B False
   C True
   D False
   E True

A fresh unstained preparation of vaginal discharge will mostly show desquamated epithelial cells and white cells although the motile *Trichomonas vaginalis* and spermatozoa may be seen. *Neisseria gonorrhoea* requires gram-staining to see the intracellular diplococci and *Candida albicans* mycelia also require staining to be visible.

107 A True
   B False
   C False
   D False
   E False

Cervical mucus in mid-cycle is affected by oestrogenic dominance. It is increased in amount, clear and thin. It exhibits spinnbarkeit being less viscous and when direct or a microscope slide shows arbonization (ferning) but red cells are not seen. It is assessed at mid-cycle in the post-coital test when surviving sperm migration is also seen.

108 A True
   B True
   C True
   D True
   E True

Progestogen-only pills work by their effect on the endomentrium and cervical mucus, but do sometimes stop ovulation. The side-effects are amenorrhoea, menorrhagia and failure as a contraceptive resulting in pregnancy. However, they are believed to be free from thrombo-embolic side-effects and are recommended for use in patients over the age of 40 years.

109 The combined oral contraceptive is associated with the following risks:
A   hepatoma
B   cervical carcinoma
C   headache in 'the week off'
D   pre-menstrual tension
E   cholestatic jaundice

110 An intra-uterine contraceptive device is associated with the following complications:
A   amenorrhea
B   salpingitis
C   cervical erosion
D   menstrual migraine
E   actinomycosis colonization

111 Amenorrhoea and galactorrhoea may be caused by
A   thyrotoxicosis
B   pituitary tumour
C   metoclopramide
D   chlorpromazine
E   combined oral contraceptive

112 The following complications are associated with total abdominal hysterectomy:
A   lymphocyst
B   bladder atony
C   divided urethra
D   vesico–vaginal fistula
E   pulmonary embolus

109 A True
  B False
  C True
  D False
  E True

The pill has a profound effect upon the liver producing cholestatic jaundice, benign (but fatal) hepatomata and occasionally carcinoma. Headaches, weight gain, depression and hypertension are the more common and less severe problems. 'Pill headaches' which typically occur in the week off can be avoided by taking the combined oral contraceptive every day, thus suppressing periods.

110 A False
  B True
  C False
  D False
  E True

The IUCD may cause menorrhagia, spotting and encourage ascending infection leading to salpingitis and tubal damage. Spores of actinomycosis are frequently found in the cytology particularly when non-copper coils are used. This rarely produces any clinical infection. Currently there is a re-appraisal of the wisdom of using an IUCD in a nulliparous patient because of the potential risk to fertility.

111 A False
  B True
  C True
  D True
  E True

Inappropriate hyperprolactinaemia will often but not always result in amenorrhoea and galactorrhea. Prolactin is normally under the inhibitory control of prolactin inhibitory factor (probably dopamine) and this is influenced by many drugs particularly phenothiazines, anti-hypertensives, hormones and anti-emetics such as metoclopramide. The syndrome may also be produced by a pituitary prolactinoma or mixed tumour which may also result in acromegaly or Cushing's disease.

112 A False
  B False
  C False
  D True
  E True

The major complications specific to this operation are damage to the urinary tract and bowel, pelvic haematoma formation and the wound infection. Leakage of urine per vaginam suggests a vesico vaginal or uretero vaginal fistula. There are also the severe problems of any operation such as anaesthetic accidents or pulmonary embolus.

113 The following are useful in the treatment of dysfunctional uterine bleeding in a 45-year-old woman:

   A   dilatation and curettage
   B   oral contraception
   C   oestrogens
   D   myomectomy
   E   prostaglandins

114 A vaginal hysterectomy

   A   is appropriate therapy for dysfunctional vaginal bleeding
   B   is appropriate therapy for CIN III
   C   is appropriate therapy for stage I endometrial carcinoma
   D   is associated with the appearance of an enterocoele
   E   should usually be combined with an anterior and posterior colporrhaphy

115 The following are acceptable operations for the treatment of stress incontinence:

   A   vaginal hysterectomy
   B   abdominal hysterectomy
   C   anterior repair
   D   colposuspension
   E   Marshall–Marchetti–Kranz operation

116 Pruritus vulvae is caused by:

   A   vulval cancer
   B   hypertrophic dystrophy
   C   strongyloides
   D   vulval intra-epithelial carcinoma
   E   candidiasis

113 A True
B False
C False
D False
E False

A curettage often helps for a short time. The birth control pill is the most effective therapy but clearly unsuitable for a woman of this age. Progestogens help as do prostaglandin synthetase inhibitors and anti-fibrinolytic agents. Hysterectomy, although a surgical procedure that one would like to avoid, at least has the advantage that it works.

114 A True
B True
C False
D True
E False

The vaginal route is ideal for access to the uterus for benign conditions whether there is an attendant prolapse or not. If there is no prolapse and no descent the operation need not be combined with a repair. The formation of an enterocoele (Pouch of Douglas hernia) should be prevented by the closure of the potential space between the utero-sacral ligaments.

115 A False
B False
C True
D True
E True

Genuine stress incontinence may be treated by the vaginal route by an anterior colporraphy or a Marchetti repair. A vaginal hysterectomy without repair will not help. Nowadays there is a move towards the abdominal route as the primary operation, particularly a Burch colposuspension, a sling procedure or Marshall–Marchetti–Kranz procedure.

116 A False
B True
C False
D True
E True

The most common causes of pruritus vulvae are trichomonas or *Candida* infections. The chronic vulval dystrophies, particularly the hypertrophic dystrophy and vulval intra-epithelial carcinoma cause pruritus, but vulval cancer causes pain rather than itching. Thread worms, not hook worms cause pruritus vulvae in children.

117 Trichomoniasis is associated with:
- **A** a white-coloured discharge
- **B** gonorrhoea
- **C** a high vaginal pH
- **D** pregnancy
- **E** antibiotic therapy

118 Which of the following associations are correct:
- **A** mittelschmerz and menorrhagia
- **B** congestive dysmenorrhoea and pelvic inflammatory disease
- **C** cystitis and menopause
- **D** pain before bleeding and ectopic pregnancy
- **E** deep dyspareunia of short duration and endometriosis

119 Ultrasonic examination in gynaecology is useful for
- **A** locating ureteric damage
- **B** identifying ovulation
- **C** identifying lost IUCD
- **D** identifying carcinoma of the endometrium
- **E** identifying a hydatidiform mole

120 Post-menopausal bleeding is caused by:
- **A** cancer of the cervix
- **B** cervical erosion
- **C** uterine fibroids
- **D** cancer of the bladder
- **E** sarcoma botryoides

117 A False
B True
C False
D False
E False

Trichomonas vaginitis is characteristically described as a profuse green frothy discharge and the white curdy discharge is the textbook (although not always correct) description of monilia. However, it is necessary to use culture in the laboratory or outpatient microscopy to clarify the diagnosis. Trichomonal infection often co-exists with gonorrhoea, but unlike monilia is not associated with pregnancy or antibiotic therapy.

118 A False
B True
C True
D True
E True

Mittelschmerz is mid-cycle ovulatory pain. The pain of chronic pelvic pathology such as pelvic inflammatory disease and endometriosis is typically congestive in type and the deep dyspareunia occurring with endometriosis lasts for many hours after the event. Atrophic cystitis occurs in the same way as atrophic vaginitis with oestrogen deficiency of the menopause. Classically pain precedes bleeding with an ectopic pregnancy and occurs after bleeding with a miscarriage.

119 A False
B True
C True
D False
E True

Ultrasonic examination has yet to find its real place in gynaecology but certainly is able to detect ovulation and even hyperstimulation of several follicles. The snow storm appearance of hydatidiform mole is characteristic. It can be used to detect ovarian tumours as a screening procedure and pelvic secondaries but it is not useful in detecting mid-line primaries.

120 A True
B False
C False
D True
E False

Post-menopausal bleeding always requires examination under anaesthesia and a diagnostic curettage. It may be due to carcinoma of the corpus, cervical polyps, atrophic vaginitis, and also a result of oestrogen therapy or maybe confused with haematuria due to carcinoma of the bladder. Uterine fibroids should involute after the menopause and sarcoma botryoides is a disease of children.

121 Dysfunctional uterine bleeding is associated with:
- **A** cervical polyp
- **B** abnormal endometrial oestrogen synthesis
- **C** high plasma FSH levels
- **D** adolescence
- **E** infertility

122 The climacteric is associated with:
- **A** irregular bleeding
- **B** vaginal dryness
- **C** headaches
- **D** insomnia
- **E** epigastric pain

123 The following statements about the climacteric are correct:
- **A** plasma FSH levels are higher than plasma LH levels
- **B** plasma triglyceride levels decrease
- **C** plasma calcium decreases
- **D** plasma testosterone is unchanged
- **E** osteoporosis can be prevented by oestrogen therapy

124 Hydatidiform moles
- **A** secrete thyroxine
- **B** secrete HCG
- **C** secrete insulin
- **D** are usually female in genotype
- **E** are associated with ovarian cysts

121 A False
    B False
    C True
    D True
    E True

Dysfunctional bleeding is defined as abnormal bleeding in the absence of tumour, inflammation or pregnancy. Hence the presence of a cervical polyp or fibroids exclude the diagnosis. It occurs commonly in the few years after puberty and preceding the menopause. The cycles are anovulatory and may have a high FSH and low progesterone levels.

122 A True
    B True
    C True
    D True
    E False

The classical vasomotor symptoms of the menopause are hot flushes, night sweats, headaches and palpitations. Vaginal dryness and loss of libido are psycho-sexual problems. Insomnia is caused by night sweats and there are numerous psychological symptoms of depression, irritability, loss of memory, lack of confidence etc. Irregular bleeding occurs and should be investigated.

123 A True
    B False
    C False
    D True
    E True

Following the cessation of periods there is a ten- to twenty-fold increase in FSH and a three-fold increase in LH. There are increased levels in triglycerides and cholesterol. The elevation of plasma calcium indicates loss of calcium from the skeleton. Osteoporosis is an important metabolic problem following ovarian failure which can almost certainly be prevented by replacement of oestrogen.

124 A False
    B True
    C False
    D True
    E True

Hydatidiform moles secrete a thyroid-stimulating substance (not thyroxine) and the patients may be thyrotoxic. They also secrete HCG which is the ideal tumour marker for future chemotherapy. Bilateral theca-lutein cysts are quite common, presumably as a result of the abundant HCG secretion from trophoblast. The great danger is malignant change to choriocarcinoma which occurs in approximately 1% of patients in Europe and 10% in the Far East.

125 Retroversion causes:
A backache
B dystocia
C dyspareunia
D anovulation
E dysmenorrhoea

126 Infertility is caused by
A Cushing's syndrome
B hyperprolactinaemia
C hypothyroidism
D Sheehan's syndrome
E Kallman's syndrome

127 The following are characteristic features of endometriosis:
A blocked tubes
B black spots
C menorrhagia
D spasmodic dysmenorrhoea
E a good symptomatic response to oestrogens

125 A True
  B False
  C True
  D False
  E False

A mobile retroversion causes few if any problems, but might be responsible for low backache and deep dyspareunia. Fixed retroversion is associated with pelvic pathology such as endometriosis or pelvic inflammatory disease, and will be associated with the pain, infertility and the more severe prolonged dyspareunia of the primary conditions.

126 A True
  B True
  C True
  D True
  E True

Kallman's syndrome is hypothalamic failure with anosmia. This causes anovulation as does the post-partum pituitary necrosis of Sheehan's syndrome. Elevated serum prolactin levels whether due to a small pituitary tumour or drug induced also stop ovulation and hypothyroidism needs to be excluded in any investigation of anovulatory infertility.

127 A False
  B True
  C True
  D False
  E False

Endometriosis is the deposition of ectopic areas of endometrium sometimes like tiny black spots on pelvic tissues particularly the utero-sacral ligaments, ovaries and peritoneal surfaces. Classical symptoms are infertility, congestive dysmenorrhea, menorrhagia, backache and dyspareunia. Treatment is surgical or by progestogens or the anti-gonadotrophin hormone danazol which produces a temporary menopause.

128 Hydatidiform mole

A occurs most frequently in S.E. Asia
B may be followed by choriocarcinoma
C is associated with follicular cysts of the ovary
D may be diagnosed at 14 weeks gestation by abdominal X-ray
E may present with excessive vomiting

129 Septic abortion

A follows spontaneous abortion
B is associated with bowel damage
C should be evacuated after the temperature has returned to normal
D should have a central venous pressure line
E is usually infected with *Clostridium welchii*

130 Monilial vaginitis

A is treated with metronidazole
B is associated with a green, frothy discharge
C is common in pregnancy
D may be asymptomatic
E characteristically has white plaques on the vaginal wall

128 A True
  B True
  C False
  D False
  E True

Hydatidiform mole is a developmental abnormality of the trophoblast. It usually presents with vaginal bleeding and the symptoms associated with pregnancy are often exaggerated. The high levels of human chorionic gonadotrophins (HCG) produced may lead to the formation of theca-lutein cysts of the ovaries. The diagnosis may be confirmed by the high levels of HCG and by a characteristic appearance on ultrasound and X-ray of the abdomen may be helpful after the eighteenth week of pregnancy.

129 A True
  B True
  C False
  D False
  E False

Sepsis may complicate any type of abortion even spontaneous abortion although it is particularly common after criminally induced abortion. In these cases retained products may be neglected and there is a high possibility of uterine or bowel damage. Anaerobic organisms are often involved and it is important to use an antibiotic regimen which will be effective against them. Evacuation of the uterus should be delayed until adequate antibiotic levels have been achieved, but not until the temperature has returned to normal. A CVP line may be necessary if there is septic shock but not for less complicated septic abortions.

130 A False
  B False
  C True
  D True
  E True

Monilial vaginitis is the most common type of lower genital tract infection found in pregnancy. It may be asymptomatic, but often causes intense vulval irritation. The textbook description of (B) is the classical description of trichomoniasis. However, there is in practice much overlap of appearance. Monilia can be treated with a local application of anti-fungal agents such as nystatin or miconazole, clotrimazole or the oral preparation Ketoconazole. Old fashioned remedies such as gentian violet may be useful when other methods are unsuccessful.

131 Spontaneous abortion

A occurs in up to 10% of all pregnancies
B is frequently due to chromosomal abnormalities
C may be prevented by giving progestogens to the mother
D may occur up to the thirtieth week of pregnancy
E may follow maternal pyrexia

132 The following procedures are performed by laparoscopy:

A Pomeroy sterilization
B tubal evaluation
C removal of a lost IUCD
D ventrosuspension
E second look for ovarian carcinoma

133 In normal sexual response

A vaginal lubrication occurs from the cervical and vulval glands
B the upper vagina dilates
C the orgasmic platform occurs in mid-vagina
D there are three stages—excitation, orgasm and resolution
E the uterus contracts with orgasm

134 Laparoscopy may reveal the following features:

A endometriosis
B ovulation
C subphrenic secondaries
D defective luteal phase
E pelvic congestion syndrome

131 A False
   B True
   C False
   D False
   E True

Spontaneous abortion occurs in up to 25% of pregnancies and is defined as the expulsion of the product of conception before the period of viability. For many countries this is taken as 28 weeks although 22 weeks (or 500 gm fetal weight) is preferable. Chromosomal abnormalities are the commonest cause of spontaneous abortion and the earlier in gestation the abortion occurs, the more likely is this to be the cause.

132 A False
   B True
   C True
   D True
   E True

The Pomeroy procedure needs a laparotomy or mini-laparotomy. Laparoscopy is commonly used for assessing infertility or the cause of pelvic pain. A lost IUCD can be retrieved and round ligaments shortened. An interim second look for ovarian carcinoma can be performed although a more extensive second look laparotomy is a better procedure.

133 A False
   B True
   C True
   D False
   E True

Vaginal lubrication comes from transudation of fluid through the vaginal wall and not from local glands. The orgasmic platform is a swelling in the outer third of the vagina occurring during excitation phase. The four stages are: excitation, plateau, orgasm and resolution and it would appear that this response is identical whether the orgasm is clitorial or vaginal.

134 A True
   B True
   C True
   D False
   E False

Laparoscopy is invaluable for the investigation of infertility and the diagnosis of pelvic pain. Although the laparoscope is inserted in the umbilicus, one can view in a cephalad direction in the search for secondaries at the time of the second look laparoscopy. Pelvic congestion syndrome may be quite common but there are no distinctive naked eye changes. The black spots of endometriosis and the stigma and corpus luteum of ovulation should be clearly seen.

135 Hirsutism
A usually has an adrenal cause
B occurs in testicular feminization
C is best treated with cyproterone acetate
D is associated with galactorrheoa
E usually has high testosterone levels

136 The following diseases occur more commonly in black patients than white patients:
A fibroids
B ectopic pregnancy
C ovarian carcinoma
D anorexia nervosa
E uterine prolapse

137 Fibroids
A are benign tumours of smooth muscle
B have distinctive ultrasonic features
C occur in the ovary
D may be visible on X-ray
E usually enlarge after the menopause

135 A False
B False
C True
D False
E False

Hirsutes may have an adrenal or an ovarian cause but in most cases it is constitutional and is not associated with any increase in plasma androgens. The rare case wih an adrenal cause can be treated with corticosteroids and occasionally suppression of ovulation helps the condition if it has an ovarian cause. However, the best treatment is by cyproterone acetate. Women with testicular feminization characteristically have scanty hair growth.

136 A True
B True
C False
D False
E False

Fibroids are very common in black patients and ectopic pregnancy is a major cause of maternal death in this group. Perhaps this is due to the increased incidence of pelvic inflammatory disease and tubal damage. Keloid formation in abdominal scars can be a problem. Ovarian carcinoma and uterine prolapse are quite rare, but cervical carcinoma is almost certainly more common in this population.

137 A True
B False
C False
D True
E False

Fibroids are benign smooth muscle tumours which become more and more replaced by fibrous tissue. They should involute and virtually disappear after the menopause but will not if they have become calcified. They may then be visible on X-ray but they do not have any characteristic ultrasonic features. Fibromas (not fibroids) may occur in the ovary.

138 Copper-containing IUCD

A should be changed every year
B have a higher incidence of actinomycosis colonization than plastic devices
C causes an increase in ectopic pregnancies
D have been implicated as a cause of fatal infection in pregnancies
E do not cause menorrhagia

139 Dyspareunia may result from:

A the climacteric
B multiparity
C adenomyosis
D granulosa cell tumour
E bromocriptine therapy

140 The following are examples of copper-containing intra-uterine devices:

A Dalkon Shield
B Multiload 250
C Lippes loop
D Progestasert
E Hodge

141 The following hormones are used in oral contraceptives:

A stilboestrol
B menstranol
C oestradiol 17 beta
D 19 nortestosterone derivatives
E progesterone

138 A False
B False
C False
D False
E False

Copper coils need to be changed every 2 or 3 years and have a lower incidence of actinomycosis colonization. They may be extruded, fail or cause menorrhagia as can any IUCD. There is much doubt whether the increased incidence of ectopics with the coil is real or relative, and whether it is primarily a result of the device.

139 A True
B False
C False
D False
E False

The atrophic vaginitis of the menopause may cause dyspareunia as may vaginal infections or endometriosis or pelvic inflammatory disease. Granulosa cell tumour secretes oestrogen and bromocriptine therapy corrects the low oestrogen levels of hyperprolactinaemia and thus should not have any deleterious effect upon intercourse.

140 A False
B True
C False
D False
E False

The Multiload copper C250, Copper 7 and Copper T are the most common copper-containing devices. The Dalkon Shield has been discontinued due to the danger of ascending infection of the braided multifilament coil. The Progestasert is a small progesterone-containing coil. The Lippes loop has been the most durable of all the plastic devices. The Hodge pessary is a weird device which some people believe relieves symptoms of retroversion.

141 A False
B True
C False
D True
E False

The oestrogen component of the pill is either mestranol or ethinyloestradiol. Many gestogens are used with a usually 19 nortestosterone derivative such as noretisterone. Pure progesterone is not used as oral absorption is poor and the half life is inadequate. Oestradiol 17 beta is also too weak in acceptable doses for ovulation suppression.

142 **Basic rules of tubal microsurgery are**
    A   the use of fine catgut
    B   the use of small abdominal incision
    C   closure of all raw peritoneal areas
    D   irrigation with isotonic solution
    E   splinting of the repaired tubes

143 **In vitro fertilization is useful treatment for**
    A   blocked tubes
    B   azospermia
    C   anti-sperm antibodies
    D   premature menopause
    E   endometriosis

144 **The following methods can be used to locate a lost IUCD:**
    A   straight AP X-ray of the pelvis
    B   ultrasound
    C   hysteroscopy
    D   geiger counter
    E   colpotomy

145 **The following instructions are appropriate for the use of a diaphragm:**
    A   remove and wash diaphragm ½ hour after intercourse
    B   sterilize before insertion
    C   always use spermicidal cream
    D   anterior ridge of diaphragm should be approximately 2 inches from pubic ramus
    E   it should be changed every 6 months

142 A False
B False
C True
D True
E False

Microsurgery often means a macroincision to ensure good exposure and gentle handling of the Fallopian tubes. In all tubal surgery fine 6/0 or 4/0 non-absorbable material such as nylon should be used. Catgut is removed through rotting and has probably ruined as many tubes as has gonorrhoea. Splinting for any length of time damages the tubal cilia and is not recommended.

143 A True
B False
C True
D False
E True

In vitro fertilization and embryo transfer into the recipient now has approximately a 10% success rate and is used principally when the tubes are blocked by infection or the tubal pick up mechanism is ineffective due to the fibrosis of endometriosis. It is also useful to overcome cervical hostility and the problems of oligospermia. Failure of ovulation or the absence of any spermatozoa cannot be helped by this technique.

144 A False
B True
C True
D False
E False

Ultrasound, hysteroscopy, curettage, laparoscopy and also the insertion of a second IUCD followed by a lateral and AP X-ray are reasonable ways of locating a lost IUCD. A straight AP X-ray is inadequate as the presence of a radio-opaque coil does not indicate whether it is in the uterine cavity or any other pelvic midline structure.

145 A False
B False
C True
D False
E False

The diaphragm is an effective method of contraception but does require considerable commitment and motivation. Spermicidal cream should always be used with it, and the diaphram should remain in place for at least 6 hr after intercourse. Fitting should be checked and the cervix should be felt to be beneath the cap and the anterior rim close to the inferior margin of the pubic ramus. The cap may last for several years but should be refitted 6 weeks after any pregnancy.

146 Ovulation can only be firmly diagnosed by pregnancy, but clinically we accept that ovulation has taken place if we find
   A   an increased luteal phase oestradiol
   B   secretory endometrium
   C   pseudo-decidual endometrium
   D   increased luteal phase prolactin
   E   stigmata of ovulation at laparoscopy

147 The following are XX genotype
   A   testicular feminization
   B   normal female
   C   pure gonadal dysgenesis
   D   hydatidiform mole
   E   polycystic ovary syndrome

148 In the investigation of infertility, it is of specific importance to question the patient about the
   A   occurrence of dysmenorrhea
   B   occurrence of dyspareunia
   C   frequency of orgasms
   D   length of menstrual cycle
   E   history of previous terminations

149 Characteristic complications of termination of early pregnancy include
   A   cornual blockage
   B   endometriosis
   C   Asherman's syndrome
   D   premature labour
   E   placental abruption

146 A False
B True
C False
D False
E True

Clinically ovulation is diagnosed by an elevation in day 21 plasma progesterone and by the finding of secretory endometrium. If laparoscopy is performed the ostium of ovulation of the corpus luteum of ovulation may be seen. Hyperprolactinaemia prevents ovulation and pseudo-decidual endometrium occurs with prolonged progestogen therapy such as taking the combined oral contraceptive.

147 A False
B True
C False
D True
E True

Patients with testicular feminization and those with pure gonadal dysgenesis (as opposed to Turner's syndrome who also have streak gonads) have an XY genotype. Hydatidiform moles are nearly always XX and women with the various syndromes which cause hirsuitism are of course always XX.

148 A True
B True
C False
D True
E True

The causes of infertility are legion and virtually every item in a gynaecological history is relevant. Deep dyspareunia and congestive dysmenorrhea suggest pathology and spasmodic dysmenorrhea, and a 28-day cycle suggests normal ovulation. Galactorrhea is associated with hyperprolactinaemia and anovulation. However the occurrence of organisms is irrelevant to fertility.

149 A True
B False
C True
D True
E False

During vaginal termination of pregnancy the fundus can be perforated, the cervix damaged and the introduction of infection may produce infertility by tubal, particularly cornual damage. Cervical incompetence may lead to mid-trimester abortion or premature labour, and removal of the decidua may lead to uterine synechiae or Asherman's syndrome with infertility and amenorrhea.

150 **Uterine enlargement may be caused by**
   A   adenomyosis
   B   pelvic inflammatory disease
   C   post-pill amenorrhoea
   D   endometriosis
   E   post-menopausal oestrogen therapy

151 **When an incomplete abortion appears in casualty, it is essential to**
   A   evacuate the uterus immediately
   B   perform a speculum examination
   C   administer ergometrine
   D   perform an ultrasonic scan
   E   cross match blood

152 **A Wertheim (radical) hysterectomy includes:**
   A   a pelvic lymphadenectomy
   B   removal of the upper third of the vagina
   C   inguinal lymphadenectomy
   D   construction of an ileal conduit
   E   radiotherapy

153 **Botryoid sarcoma**
   A   usually occurs in childhood
   B   is a rhabdomyosarcoma
   C   produces a tumour marker
   D   is not sensitive to chemotherapy
   E   is a tumour of the uterine body.

150 A True
B False
C False
D False
E True

The principle causes of uterine enlargement are pregnancy, fibroids and adenomyosis although oestrogen replacement therapy is fast becoming an important cause of uterine pathology and enlargement. Pelvic inflammatory disease and (external) endometriosis cause similar clinical pictures of pelvic pain and dyspareunia but the uterus is not enlarged. Post-pill amenorrhoea is associated with a small uterus.

151 A False
B True
C True
D False
E False

An incomplete abortion is the most common of all gynaecological emergencies. It is necessary to stop bleeding and evacuate the uterus. Ergometrine should be given and a speculum examination may reveal products within the cervix which can be removed with sponge-holding forceps. A formal evacuation can wait until a convenient time and cross matching blood or use of ultrasound is a wasteful misuse of facilities and technology.

152 A True
B True
C False
D False
E False

A Wertheim hysterectomy is performed for carcinoma of the cervix and also for stage II carcinoma of corpus as this involves the cervix. It is an abdominl hysterectomy with bilateral salpingo-oophoectomy removing the iliac, pre-sacral and obturator nodes and the upper third of the vagina. Radiotherapy is not part of the procedure, but may be added for overall treatment of the disease.

153 A True
B True
C False
D False
E False

Botryoid sarcoma appears as the fungating grape-like tumour from the vagina or cervix in young girls. It was thought to be a mixed mesodermal tumour, but it is now accepted as a rhabdomyosarcoma. It is sensitive to chemotherapy and radiotherapy, but unfortunately radical surgery is often still required to improve the prognosis.

154 A choriocarcinoma may present by:

A breathlessness
B a breast lump
C a suburethral mass
D a stroke
E the passage of 'vesicles'

155 Malignant changes which occur in the vulva include:

A hyperplastic dystrophy
B Bechet's syndrome
C Paget's disease
D lichen schlerosis
E melanoma

156 Stage IB cervical cancer:

A is pre-invasive
B is usually adenocarcinoma
C is treated by total abdominal hysterectomy
D is associated with deep pelvic pain
E can be diagnosed by colposcopy

157 CIN III

A includes severe dysplasia
B is usually cured by a cone biopsy
C has node involvement in approximately 2% of cases
D may involve the vaginal vault
E commences as squamous metaplasia

154 A True
B False
C True
D True
E False

Choriocarcinoma may present with an abdominal mass or pain together with vaginal bleeding. Passage of vesicles occurs with a mole. Metastatic manifestations which are often the presenting symptoms include a suburethral mass typically purple in colour, breathlessness, haemoptysis or a cerebrovascular accident.

155 A False
B False
C True
D False
E True

Malignant tumours which occur in the vulva include squamous carcinoma, basal cell carcinoma, Paget's disease and melanoma. There are many pre-malignant hyperplastic conditions which were until recently called leucoplakia and also a bunch of odd eponymous terms. They are now referred to as a group—hyperplastic dystrophy or vulval intra-epithelial neoplasia (VIN III).

156 A False
B False
C False
D False
E False

Stage IB cervical cancer is invasive and confined to the cervix. 95% are squamous in type and 5% adenocarcinoma. This early stage is usually asymptomatic or has trivial symptoms of irregular bleeding which are tragically ignored. The diagnosis cannot be made without biopsy. Treatment is by a Wertheim hysterectomy with or without radium or external radiotherapy.

157 A True
B True
C False
D True
E False

Cervical intra-epithelial neoplasia (CIN) III is either severe dysplasia or carcinoma in situ. It is nearly always cured by a cone biopsy, following colposcopy. It is not malignant and therefore there will be no node involvement. The pathology starts at the squama-columnar junction and may involve the tissue laterally to the vaginal vaults.

158 Diethylstilboestrol (DES) exposure in utero is associated with:
   A   clear cell carcinoma of the vagina
   B   ovarian carcinoma
   C   Brenner tumour
   D   vaginal adenosis
   E   cervical hoods

159 Cancer of the endometrium occurs more commonly in association with:
   A   obesity
   B   progestogen therapy
   C   infertility
   D   late menopause
   E   oral contraception

160 Endometrial carcinoma is:
   A   usually adenocarcinoma
   B   more frequent with high parity
   C   more frequent in association with an ovarian fibroma
   D   a more dangerous tumour than ovarian carcinoma
   E   more common with combined oral contraceptive

158 A True
B False
C False
D True
E True

Young women who are needlessly exposed in utero to diethylstilboestrol are at considerable risk of developing vaginal adenosis and a very small risk of developing clear cell carcinoma of the vagina. Cervical hoods and cockscombs are also a feature. These women need skilled long term colposcopic follow-up. Radical surgery should be avoided unless malignancy occurs.

159 A True
B False
C True
D True
E False

Endometrial carcinoma has a strong association with obesity, infertility due to anovulation, late menopause, granulosa and theca cell tumours, Stein–Leventhal syndrome and unopposed oestrogen therapy in post-menopausal women. The common denominator in these conditions is the continuous stimulation with oestrogen without the monthly anti-proliferative effect of progesterone (or progestogen). Carcinoma of the endometrium is thus less common in patients having the combined oral contraceptive pill and can be prevented in the post-menopausal woman by the addition of progestogen to any oestrogen therapy that she may be receiving.

160 A True
B False
C False
D False
E False

Endometrial carcinoma is more common in infertile women, particularly with anovulation, and is certainly less common in patients with high parity. It is also more common with functioning ovarian tumours but the fibroma does not secrete oestrogens. It is less common with the combined oral contraceptive because of the antiproliferative effect of progestogen.

161 The following ovarian tumours are malignant:
A   Brenner tumour
B   dermoid cyst
C   Krukenberg tumour
D   granulosa cell tumour
E   endodermal sinus tumour

162 Micro-invasive cancer of the cervix
A   is stage I A
B   is squamous carcinoma
C   has lymph node involvement in 5%
D   is curable by cone biopsy
E   can be diagnosed by colposcopy

163 The following statements about cervical cytology are correct:
A   screening programmes have not resulted in a decrease in mortality from cancer
B   dyskaryosis frequently reverts to normal cytology
C   malignant cells have a decreased nuclear/cytoplasmic ratio
D   screening should begin at age 30 years
E   a grade V smear indicates malignancy

164 The following statements about carcinoma of the ovary are appropriate:
A   more women die of ovarian cancer than uterine and cervix combined
B   the omentum should be removed at the initial laparotomy
C   subphrenic deposits indicate stage II disease
D   Cis-platinum treatment is complicated by renal failure
E   the disease is associated with high parity

161 A False
B False
C True
D True
E True

Brenner tumours and dermoid cysts are benign, but the latter has a malignant form in a malignant teratoma. The endodermal sinus tumour is a rare germ cell tumour of high malignancy which is of great interest because it secretes HCG and AFP. These are effective tumour markers for chemotherapy. Granulosa cell tumours may recur 20 years after the primary, and Krukenberg tumours are secondary.

162 A True
B True
C False
D True
E False

Microinvasive carcinoma has passed through the basement membrane to a depth of up to 3 mm into the stroma of the cervix. It is a difficult tissue diagnosis rather than one made by colposcopy. It very rarely (1–2%) has a lymph node involvement and therefore can be usually cured by cone biopsy if the margins are free of disease.

163 A False
B True
C False
D False
E False

It is true that the benefits of mass screening programmes have been slow to emerge, but the benefits are now well accepted particularly in an age of greater sexual contact, venereal disease and cervical cancer in young women. Malignant cells have an increase in nuclear/cytoplasmic ratio but these features must not be taken as diagnostic of malignancy as a cone or a colposcopically directed punch biopsy is necessary for a tissue diagnosis.

164 A True
B True
C False
D True
E False

Ovarian carcinoma is so often at an advanced stage when recognized that its overall prognosis is poor. The initial staging laparotomy is an extensive procedure with removal of the uterus, both ovaries, omentum and a thorough search for metastatic deposits, including the liver and under the diaphragm. Subphrenic deposits indicate stage III disease and the need for chemotherapy, nowadays in the form of Cis-platinum.

165 Stein–Leventhal syndrome is associated with:
A oligomenorrhea
B cancer of the breast
C anorexia nervosa
D abnormality of adrenal function
E ovarian malignancy

166 Cancer of the vagina is:
A a squamous carcinoma
B approximately as common as vulval carcinoma
C associated with prolonged use of a ring pessary
D radiosensitive
E treated by a Shauta operation

167 A dilatation and curettage is useful in:
A diagnosis of endometriosis
B treatment of fibroids
C diagnosis of pelvic tuberculosis
D treatment of congestive dysmenorrhoea
E diagnosis of hyperprolactinaemia

168 The following tumours are sensitive to chemotherapy:
A cancer of the vulva
B cancer of the cervix
C cancer of the ovary
D choriocarcinoma
E dysgerminoma

165 A True
B False
C False
D True
E False

Stein–Leventhal syndrome or the polycystic ovary syndrome is manifested by oligomenorrhea or anemorrhea, obesity, hirsutism and infertility. There is an association with cancer of the endometrium but not with the breast. It is probably due basically to abnormality of adrenal function which produces polycystic changes and hyperthecosis in the ovaries. Ovulation induction can usually be achieved by clomiphene. The former use of wedge resection of the ovaries is now a thing of the past as it often caused severe fimbrial adhesions.

166 A True
B False
C True
D True
E False

Squamous cancer of the vagina is a rare tumour occurring after the menopause. It is moderately radiosensitive but not sensitive to chemotherapy. Treatment is a combination of radiotherapy and radical surgery, but not by a Shauta procedure which is an obsolete vaginal operation for cancer of the cervix.

167 A False
B False
C True
D False
E False

A curettage is essentially a diagnostic procedure and is not really effective with any treatment except perhaps in dysfunctional uterine bleeding, primary spasmodic dysmenorrhoea or removal of an endometrial polyp. Endometrial biopsy may help diagnose pelvic tuberculosis or anovulation.

168 A False
B False
C True
D True
E True

Chemotherapy is not helpful for most gynaecological cancers. Progestogen is of doubtful value for endometrium cancer. Cis-platinum has recently given some hope for ovarian carcinoma either used as a single agent or in combination. Major advances have been made in the treatment of choriocarcinoma and the rare germ cell tumours, dysgerminoma and endodermal sinus tumour in association with tumour markers.

169 A pleural effusion characteristically occurs with:

   A   cancer of the cervix

   B   cancer of the ovary

   C   benign ovarian fibroma

   D   mixed mesodermal tumour

   E   Hydatid of Morgani

169 A False
B True
C True
D True
E False

Cervical squamous carcinoma tends to remain within the pelvis and not have distant metastasis. On the other hand cancer of the ovary and a mixed mesodermal tumour of the ovary have lung secondaries and pleural effusions. The benign ovarian fibroma produces a syndrome of ascites and pleural effusion (Meigs syndrome—first described by Lawson Tait). The Hydatid of Morgani is a benign Woolfian duct remnant.

CASE HISTORY

A 60-year-old patient reports a recent heavy 3-day bleed. Examination reveals a healthy woman with a mobile normal size uterus and a small cervical polyp with atrophic vaginitis.

170 It would be correct to:
- **A** remove polyp and await histology
- **B** prescribe oestrogen vaginal cream
- **C** admit for dilatation and curettage and polypectomy
- **D** enquire about oestrogen therapy
- **E** perform a vabra curettage

The polyp is benign and the fractional curettage reveals a normal endocervix, but a well-differentiated cancer of the corpus.

171 The tumour is:
- **A** most likely to be adenocarcinoma
- **B** stage I
- **C** grade II
- **D** has a 5-year prognosis in excess of 80%
- **E** probably due to exogenous oestrogen therapy

There are several acceptable methods of treating this patient.

172 These include:
- **A** progestogen therapy
- **B** intra-cavity radium
- **C** a vaginal hysterectomy
- **D** abdominal hysterectomy and radium
- **E** a Wertheim hysterectomy

The hysterectomy specimen reveals that the tumour has invaded the myometrium almost to the serosal surface.

173 Which of the following statements are correct:
- **A** the tumour is really stage I
- **B** the patient need post-operative radiotherapy
- **C** the patient needs cytoxics
- **D** the prognosis is adversely influenced by the myometrial invasion
- **E** lymph node secondaries will be found in 50% of patients

170 A False
    B False
    C True
    D True
    E False

Although the patient has atrophic vaginitis and a cervical polyp, it is wrong to assume either of these as being the cause of post-menopausal bleeding. The patient must have a curettage before any other treatment is considered. This curettage should be under anaesthesia, as an in-patient. Vabra is not thorough enough in the post-menopausal patient who has a tight cervix and a very high probability of intra-uterine malignancy.

171 A True
    B True
    C False
    D True
    E False

This well-differentiated tumour localized to the corpus is stage I, grade I with a 95% chance that it is an adenocarcinoma. Its prognosis is good. Although unopposed oestrogens cause endometrial carcinoma, this patient has atrophic vaginitis and a normal size uterus and there is no reason to suspect this as an aetiological factor.

172 A False
    B False
    C False
    D True
    E False

As the cervix is not involved there is no need for a radical Wertheim hysterectomy with node dissection. However, it is important to take the adnexae and, in order to prevent a vault recurrence, either remove the cuff of vagina or give post-operative vault radium. A vaginal hysterectomy is inadequate and progestogen will not work. Intra-cavity radium is unnecessary and ruins the specimen for consideration of depth of myometrial invasion although it could be justified in sick patients who have a high anaesthetic risk.

173 A False
    B True
    C False
    D True
    E False

One of the problems of the current staging system is that it does not consider the depth of invasion although this is a major prognostic factor. The tumour is still stage I. The patient needs vault radium or external radiotherapy but cytotoxic therapy is not helpful. Lymph node involvement occurs in 10% of stage I tumours and it will be increased to 25% with increased myometrial invasion.

CASE HISTORY

A young 19-year-old unmarried girl presents at Gynaecology out-patients with a profuse irritant malodourous vaginal discharge.

174 Which of the following points in the history may specifically help clarify this diagnosis:
- **A** date of last menstrual period
- **B** history of recent coitus
- **C** type of birth control
- **D** details of employment
- **E** any history of previous termination of pregnancy

175 What findings on examination might co-exist with this condition:
- **A** adnexal tenderness
- **B** cervical ectopy
- **C** positive cervical cytology
- **D** tender nodularity of the utero-sacral ligaments
- **E** fixed retroversion

176 Gram-staining of the discharge may show:
- **A** monilia
- **B** chlamydia
- **C** mycoplasma
- **D** gram-positive intracellular diplococci
- **E** *Trichomonas vaginalis*

Microscopy and/or culture reveals the presence of *Trichomonas vaginalis* and gonorrhoea

177 Which of the following statements are correct:
- **A** serology helps assess response to treatment
- **B** Metronidazole 200 mg daily is first line treatment of *Trichomonas vaginalis*
- **C** Procaine penicillin is first-line treatment of gonorrhea
- **D** salpingitis may occur in approximately 40% of patients
- **E** contacts should be sought and treated

174 **A** False
  B True
  C True
  D False
  E False

Such a vaginal discharge is often related to sexual intercourse. It could be related to non-barrier methods of contraception and the pill may predispose to monilial vaginitis. Although professionals may be more at risk from vaginal or venereal infections no group is immune to this problem.

175 **A** True
  B False
  C True
  D False
  E True

Adnexal tenderness and swelling together with fixed retroversion are characteristic findings in subacute or chronic pelvic inflammatory disease. There will be a greater incidence of positive cytology. Utero-sacral nodularity is a feature of endometriosis and cervical ectopy is not related to infection but is due to the exposure of endocervical columnar epithelium.

176 **A** True
  B False
  C False
  D False
  E True

Gram-staining may show monilia, trichomonads, the gram-negative intracellular diplococci of gonorrhea, gram-negative organisms of *Gardenerella* and also profuse numbers of white and red blood cells. The pus cells and trichomonads will also be visible in a simple unstained saline preparation.

177 **A** False
  B False
  C True
  D False
  E True

Metronidazole 200 mg t.d.s. will eradicate most cases of trichomoniasis and procaine penicillin is still effective in most European or African strains of gonococcus. However, resistance is becoming increasingly common particularly from the Far East and spectinomycin should be used for these cases. Co-existent chlamydia will require tetracycline or erythromycin for eradication.

OBSTETRICS

178 The following statements concerning fertilization are correct:
A   it takes place in the Fallopian tube
B   the spermatozoon has a haploid number chromosomes
C   the eight cell stage is the morula
D   the zona pellucida persists until blastocyst formation
E   telophase follows metaphase

179 The following statements about hormonal secretion in pregnancy are correct:
A   maximal HCG levels are found between days 60 and 80 of pregnancy
B   HPL raises maternal blood sugar
C   oestradiol accounts for 90% of oestrogen secreted in pregnancy
D   progesterone levels decrease before labour
E   SP1 has an ovarian origin.

180 The normal endocrinological changes occurring in pregnancy are an:
A   increased ACTH
B   increased prolactin
C   increased thyroxine levels
D   increased cortisol levels
E   increased renin levels

181 The following changes in the genital tract occur during pregnancy:
A   decreased vaginal pH
B   cervical ectopy
C   trophoblastic invasion of spiral arteries
D   the lower segment forms in the mid-trimester
E   hyperplasia and hypertrophy of myometrial fibres occur

178 A True
B True
C False
D True
E True

Fertilization occurs in the ampulla of the Fallopian tube. Within the ovarian cytoplasm the male pronucleus (haploid) joins the haploid female pronucleus after telophase. Within 3 days the morula, a solid mass of uniform cells is formed. This becomes cystic, loses the zona pelucida leaving the cells in contact with the decidua which then becomes the early placenta.

179 A True
B True
C False
D True
E False

HPL has a profound effect on lipid and the carbohydrate metabolism, but exerts a glucose-saving effect on the mother and tends to elevate blood glucose levels. SP1 is a pregnancy-specific hormone which almost certainly originates from the placenta. Its function is unknown. The principal pregnancy oestrogen is oestriol which together with progesterone increases in concentration until term. There is a fall in progesterone during the hours before labour begins.

180 A True
B True
C True
D True
E True

There is a great increase in all of these hormones, although here is no clinical evidence that pregnant women become cushingoid or thyrotoxic. However, normal values for adrenal and thyroid functions are altered in pregnancy and the diagnosis and control of hyperthyroidism, for example, may be difficult.

181 A True
B True
C True
D False
E True

The uterine weight increases from 50 to 1000 g at term and the lower segment forms only in the last 10 weeks. Trophoblastic invasion is the probable cause of the dilatation of the spiral arteries of the uterus, thus establishing a huge blood supply to the intervillous space. Increased oestrogens produce the ectopy of the cervix and the more acidic vaginal discharge.

182 The following biochemical changes occur in normal pregnancy:

A decrease in serum albumin
B decrease in serum IgG
C decrease in blood urea
D decrease in iron binding capacity
E decrease in total haemoglobin

183 The following changes in renal function occur during pregnancy:

A renal plasma flow is raised
B glomerular filtration rate increases to about 170 ml/min
C the renal pelvis dilates
D plasma renin concentration fails
E uric acid clearance increases

184 These methods of placental transfer are appropriate for the following substances:

A oxygen—active
B fats—pinocytosis
C iron—active
D carbon dioxide—passive
E antibodies—pinocytosis

185 The functions of the placenta include:

A production of erythocytes
B the formation of an immunological barrier
C excretion of waste products
D production of insulin
E production of progesterone

182 A True
  B True
  C True
  D False
  E False

There is a decreased serum albumin and IgG (which also occurs with the combined oral contraceptive) which is partly due to the haemodilution of pregnancy. This is also responsible for the decrease in haemoglobin concentration and serum iron although there is an increase in total haemoglobin and in plasma transferrin concentration. The decrease in urea and creatinine follows the 40% increase in glomerular filtration rate.

183 A True
  B True
  C True
  D False
  E True

Both renal plasma flow and glomerular filtration rate increase during pregnancy. The upper renal tract dilates and this effect is primarily mechanical although increased levels of progesterone may also be responsible. Plasma renin concentration rises markedly in the first trimester, but falls thereafter.

184 A False
  B False
  C True
  D True
  E True

Placental transfer of water, oxygen, carbon dioxide urea, sodium, and potassium is by passive methods. There is active transfer of carbohydrates, amino acids and a few proteins. IgG is transferred actively by pinocytosis.

185 A False
  B True
  C True
  D False
  E True

The placenta has immense respiratory, nutrient, excretory, endocrine and immunological functions. The success of the placenta and fetus as a homograph containing paternal antigens remains a mystery. It is possible that trophoblastic cells are immunologically inert or that there is a protective layer which separates placental antigens from maternal lymphocytes.

186 The following statements about placental pathology are appropriate:
A placenta extrachorialis predisposes to post-partum haemorrhage
B a velamentous insertion of the cord is of no clinical importance
C placenta succenturiata (a succenturiate lobe) predisposes to ante-partum haemorrhage
D a haemangioma of the placenta causes oligohydramnios
E placenta percreta penetrates through to the serosal surface of the uterus

187 In the human feto-placental unit:
A the intervillous space contains fetal blood
B the invasion of maternal spiral arteries by trophoblast causes dilatation
C two-cell membranes separate the maternal and fetal circulations
D the spiral arteries enter the placental cotyledons
E cytotrophoblast cells disappear towards term

188 The fetal circulatory changes that occur after birth are:
A rise in IVC pressure
B fall in pulmonary vascular resistance
C decrease in heart rate
D fall of right atrial pressure
E left to right shunt through the ductus arteriosus

189 The following statements about fetal physiology are correct:
A the fetal heart rate varies between 70 and 110 beats/min
B the haemoglobin concentration is 18 g/100 ml
C glycogen stores in skeletal muscle can be mobilized in the event of hypoxia
D the ductus venosus enters the inferior vena cava
E blood flows from the right to the left atrium through the foramen ovale.

186 A False
B False
C False
D False
E True

Placenta extrachorialis (marginata or circumvalata) is of little clinical significance but may predispose to an ante-partum haemorrhage. A velamentous insertion with vessels running through the membranes may result in vasa praevia or compression of the cord. A succenturiate lobe may cause a retained lobe or post-partum haemorrhage and the rare haemangioma of the placenta causes severe polyhydramnios.

187 A False
B True
C False
D False
E True

Placental blood passes through the dilated spiral arteries and flows in a pulsatile way into the inter-villous space. It cascades over the tree-like villi of the fetal cotyledons and emerges through the maternal veins. The human haemochorial placenta has the maternal blood of the intervillous space separated from the fetal blood in the terminal villi by a single later of trophoblast cells.

188 A False
B True
C True
D True
E True

With ligation of the umbilical cord there is a fall in IVC pressure which causes the ductus venosus to close; and also a fall in right atrial pressure which closes the foramen ovale. Pulmonary arterial resistance and pressure falls and the ductus arteriosus shunt becomes left to right until it is closed by muscular contractions following the rise in oxygen tension.

189 A False
B True
C False
D True
E True

Oxygenated blood (80% saturated) from the umbilical vein is mostly shunted past the liver through the ductus venosus to the inferior vena cava and the right atrium of the heart where it is joined by blood from the SVC. 75% of this is deflected through the foramen ovale to the left atrium where it is pumped to the aorta. Glycogen stores are mobilized from the liver and heart muscle but not from skeletal muscle. The normal fetal heart rate is 120 to 160.

190 The following conditions frequently improve during pregnancy:
A   iron deficiency anaemia
B   asthma
C   regional ileitis
D   depression
E   mitral stenosis

191 Immunological slide pregnancy tests
A   are positive 3 days after the expected date of the first missed period
B   depend on chorionic gonadotrophins
C   become negative if the corpus luteum is removed
D   are strongly positive in cases with hydatidiform moles
E   in normal pregnancy reach peak levels at term

192 A lateral X-ray of the pelvis in pregnancy provides information about:
A   bispinous diameter
B   subpubic arch
C   shape of the pelvic brim
D   sacral curve
E   true conjugate

193 The normal gynaecoid pelvis:
A   has a transverse brim diameter of 13 cm
B   has an angle of inclination approximately 90°
C   has a pubo-sacral diameter of 11 cm
D   encourages engagement in the transverse position
E   has a narrower fore pelvis than the android pelvis

190 A False
B True
C True
D True
E False

A greater demand for iron stores and increased plasma volume of pregnancy usually cause worsening of iron deficiency anaemia and the symptoms of mitral stenosis. It is possible that the increased maternal levels of cortisone improve conditions which are characteristically steroid responsive. Strangely depression is often better in pregnancy and suicide is rare.

191 A False
B True
C False
D True
E False

Immunological pregnancy tests such as latex precipitation become positive about 2 weeks after the first missed period. They depend on the presence of chorionic gonadotrophins and the test usually becomes negative at about 18 weeks when the HCG levels are falling. The test is strongly positive in trophoblastic disease and twins. A radioimmunoassay of the serum Beta subunit of HCG is now the most precise method available.

192 A False
B False
C False
D True
E True

An erect lateral pelvimetry is nowadays only used to assess mode of delivery for a breech presentation or possibly to assess the wisdom of vaginal delivery after previous Caesarean section. The lateral X-ray gives information about the antero-posterior diameters of the inlet, mid-cavity and the outlet.

193 A True
B False
C False
D True
E False

The gynaecoid pelvis is the ideal obstetric pelvis and contrasts significantly with the android which is the worst of the four classical pelvic types — the other two are platypelloid and anthropoid. The maximum inlet diameter is the transverse, is 13 cm and hence engagement in the transverse position is usual. Rotation occurs with descent and the head is delivered in antero-posterior plane as the pubosacral diameter is the largest diameter of the outlet at 13 cm.

194 The lower segment of the uterus

A develops in the first trimester
B contains a greater proportion of muscle fibre than the upper segment
C is separated from the upper segment at the level of reflection of the pelvic peritoneum
D is incised during a classical Caesarean section
E contains no muscle fibres

195 An incompetent cervix

A is congenital in some cases
B follows termination of pregnancy
C classically causes recurrent first trimester abortions
D should be managed with cervical cerclage
E follows a cone biopsy of the cervix

196 The following figures are approximately true for developed countries:

A the perinatal mortality rate is 15/1000 births
B the maternal death rate is 0.5/1000 births
C the neonatal death rate is 10/1000 live births
D the stillbirth rate is 20/1000 births
E 70% of infant deaths occur in the neonatal period

197 An itchy vaginal discharge in pregnancy

A is physiological
B is associated with monilial infection
C is usually psychosomatic
D is associated with amnionitis
E is associated with *Trichomonas vaginalis* infection

194 A False
B False
C True
D False
E False

The lower uterine segment develops during the last trimester. It is much thinner than the upper segment and is separated from it by the physiological ring of Bandl. The lower proportion of muscle fibres in the lower segment make its contractions less efficient and is one of the reasons for the increased incidence of post-partum haemorrhage in placenta praevia.

195 A True
B True
C False
D True
E True

Incompetent cervix may follow damage to the cervix at delivery, or following surgical procedures, but in about a third of cases there is no previous injury to account for the problem. Classically there is a history of recurrent abortions after week 14 of pregnancy. The diagnosis is confirmed by the discovery of a dilating cervix and the appropriate treatment is to perform a cervical cerclage using the Shirodkar or McDonald technique.

196 A True
B False
C True
D False
E True

The maternal death rate in developed countries is now less than 0.2/1000 total births. Perinatal mortality included stillbirths and first week neonatal deaths. The stillbirth rate is about 10/1000 births with the perinatal mortality rate about 15/1000 births. It is important for those working in the obstetric field to have knowledge of the perinatal and maternal mortality rate for their own countries or areas. The rates for developing countries are generally much higher than those for developed countries.

197 A False
B True
C False
D False
E True

Lower genital tract infections are common in pregnancy particularly monilial vaginitis following the change in local pH and trichomonas as this is a sexually transmitted disease. Any patient complaining of such an irritant discharge should be examined with a speculum and a swab taken for microscopy and culture. Upper genital tract infection is not usually associated with vulval itching nor is physiological discharge or psychoneurotic disorders.

198 Which of the following statements about the fetal skull are appropriate:

    A   suboccipito-bregmatic diameter presents with deflexion

    B   occipito-frontal diameter occurs with a posterior position

    C   submento-bregmatic diameter is 11–12 cm

    D   the bi-parietal diameter has the same diameter as the occipito-frontal

    E   the mento-vertical diameter presents in a face presentation

199 An ideal pelvis has

    A   a straight sacrum

    B   an angle of inclination of 135°

    C   a subpubic angle of about 70°

    D   a palpable sacral promontory

    E   parallel pelvic side walls

200 Amniotic fluid

    A   is bacteriocidal

    B   has a turnover of 24 hr

    C   is a nutrient

    D   is increased in fetal nephrosis

    E   prevents dessication

201 Polyhydramnios is caused by

    A   a tracheo-oesophageal fistula

    B   renal agenesis

    C   twins

    D   hydatidiform mole

    E   closed spina bifida

198 A False
B True
C False
D False
E False

The bi-parietal diameter (9.5 cm) is the transverse diameter presenting in a cephalic presentation. In a well-flexed head the suboccipito-bregmatic (9.5 cm) presents. With a posterior position deflexion occurs and the occipito-frontal diameter of 11–12 cm is found. The mento-vertical (14.0 cm) occurs in a brow presentation. The submento-bregmatic is 9.5 cm and is found with a face presentation.

199 A False
B True
C False
D False
E True

The ideal pelvis is a large gynaecoid type. It will have an angle of inclination of about 135° but this is characteristically larger in black patients hence the delay of engagement of the head. The brim is round and the sacral promontory cannot be felt. Mid-cavity qualities are straight pelvic side walls, a smooth concave sacrum and ischial spines which are not prominent. The subpubic arch should be 90°.

200 A True
B False
C True
D False
E True

Amniotic fluid has a rapid turnover every 4–6 hr, is bacteriocidal and also acts as a nutrient, a protective cushion and fundamentally as in all animals whether they are mammals, fishes, reptiles or birds develop in water its function is to prevent dessication of the growing embryo.

201 A True
B False
C True
D False
E False

Polyhydramnios occurs when there is a change in either secretion of amniotic fluid or its re-absorption by fetal swallowing. The former occurs in twins, diabetes, fetal nephrotic syndrome and from the exposed choroidal plexus of anencephaly or open spina bifida. Any alimentary obstruction such as a tracheo-oesophageal fistula or duodenal atresia will reduce re-absorption.

202 Premature rupture of the membranes at less than 34 weeks' gestation
A   is managed conservatively
B   is diagnosed on history alone
C   should usually be treated with antibiotics
D   should be allowed to labour if contractions occur
E   is caused by placenta praevia

203 The anterior fontanelle
A   is triangular shaped
B   presents in a well-flexed cephalic presentation
C   is bounded by frontal and parietal bones
D   is at the junction of the sagittal and lambdoidal sutures
E   allows moulding to occur in labour

204 The following investigations should be performed routinely at the first antenatal visit:
A   haemoglobin level
B   blood sugar
C   blood group
D   serum alpha-fetoprotein
E   serum urate

202 A True
B False
C False
D True
E False

Premature rupture of the membranes can be treated conservatively before 34 weeks' gestation provided there is no evidence of infection. A vaginal digital examination is prohibited. Prophylactic antibiotics are not helpful. A sterile speculum examination should always be done to confirm the diagnosis as the fluid loss may be urine or a vaginal discharge. It is also an opportunity to take swabs for culture, although the organisms did not always correlate with those found in the amniotic fluid with chorio-amnionitis.

203 A False
B False
C True
D False
E True

The anterior fontanelle (bregma) is the large diamond-shaped depression which occurs at the junction of the sagittal, frontal and coronal sutures. It is bounded by the parietal and frontal bones. It allows for moulding in labour and for skull growth after birth. The finding of the anterior fontanelle at vaginal examination usually means deflection and of course a larger cephalic diameter presenting to the pelvis.

204 A True
B False
C True
D False
E False

It is important to measure the haemoglobin level and determine the blood group of all patients at their first antenatal visit, as well as performing a serological test for syphilis and serology for TORCH infections (toxoplasmosis, rubella, cytomegalic virus, herpes) if they are available. Screening for neural tube defects by serum alpha-fetoprotein is only useful at 16–18 weeks with the pregnancy accurately dated by ultrasound. A test of blood sugar could be useful for specific reasons but not as a routine, and an estimation of the serum urate is of little use for anything.

205 Hyperemesis gravidarum

A usually occurs in the first trimester
B is associated with hydatidiform mole
C causes polyneuritis
D occurs most commonly in grand multigravidae
E causes jaundice

206 Acute pyelonephritis

A complicates 5% of pregnancies
B is usually caused by *E. coli*
C usually presents with urinary symptoms
D may cause a placental abruption
E treatment should be started immediately following a microscopy diagnosis

207 A patient with haemoglobin level at 9.0 g/dL at 32 weeks' gestation

A should be transfused
B should have a marrow biopsy
C probably has a physiological anaemia
D needs an intravenous infusion of iron
E is likely to have an iron deficiency anaemia

205 A True
  B True
  C True
  D False
  E True

Hyperemesis gravidarum is severe vomiting in pregnancy, usually occurring in the first trimester and in primigravid patients. It is also more common in patients with hydatidiform mole or multiple pregnancy which is probably a maternal response to excessive production of trophoblastic hormones. Untreated hyperemesis may lead to polyneuritis, liver failure and renal damage. The patient (like Charlotte Brontë) may die. It is important to exclude other causes of vomiting such as acute pyelonephritis, acute appendicitis and preicteric hepatitis.

206 A False
  B True
  C False
  D False
  E True

Acute pyelonephritis complicates 1–2% of pregnancies, is a severe disease causing abdominal pain, vomiting and rigors. It commonly has no symptoms referrable to the urinary tract such as haematuria frequency or dysuria. The urine should be examined by microscopy and the finding of organisms and white cells indicate the diagnosis and the need for chemotherapy, which can be modified if inappropriate sensitivities turn up. The finding of a normal urine on microscopy is equally important as this indicates a need to search for another possible 'surgical' cause of abdominal pain and vomiting.

207 A False
  B False
  C False
  D False
  E True

Any patient with a haemoglobin level less than 10 g/dL should be investigated but taking a sternal marrow biopsy is going too far. This level of haemoglobin is most commonly due to iron deficiency anaemia from a deficient diet, deficient iron stores or chronic blood loss. Blood transfusion and an intravenous iron infusion should be avoided as anaemia can usually be corrected by the appropriate haematinics

208 Chronic hypertension in pregnancy is associated with:
   A asymmetrical growth retardation
   B eclampsia
   C placenta praevia
   D fetal distress in labour
   E asymptomatic bacteriuria

209 Fetal distress is manifested by
   A macrosomia
   B increased fetal movement
   C increased fetal respiration
   D increased beat-to-beat variation
   E oligohydramnios

210 An 18-week ultrasound scan can:
   A distinguish sex
   B measure cerebral ventricles
   C recognize neural tube defects
   D recognize microcephaly
   E recognize duodenal atresia

211 A single ultrasound scan at 34 weeks can:
   A clarify dates
   B diagnose symmetrical growth retardation
   C diagnose anencephaly
   D diagnose fetal ascites
   E diagnose Down's syndrome

208 A True
B True
C False
D True
E True

Hypertension whether acute or chronic of any origin may produce convulsions, placental abruption, or more commonly problems of placental insufficiency. These manifestations of hypertension are asymmetric growth retardation, intra-uterine death and fetal distress in pregnancy or in labour. Asymptomatic bacteriuria is associated with chronic renal disease and chronic hypertension.

209 A False
B False
C False
D False
E True

Fetal distress reveals itself by decreased fetal movements, a poorly responsive trace and decreased beat-to-beat variation. There is often oligohydramios and sometimes growth retardation. Before labour, antenatal cardiotocography, kick counts and serial ultrasonic estimations of abdominal girth and head circumference are the best methods of assessing fetal health. Unfortunately fetal respiratory movements are not helpful in assessing the health of a high risk pregnancy.

210 A True
B True
C True
D False
E False

A full anomaly scan at 16 to 18 weeks is a vital part of contemporary obstetric care. It is possible to recognize hydrocephalus by enlarged cerebral ventricles, diagnose anencephaly and other neural tube defects. The kidneys can be outlined, as can the bladder, and congenital heart disease diagnosed. Microcephaly is much more difficult to diagnose, requiring serial measurements later in pregnancy, and duodenal atresia is diagnosed later.

211 A False
B False
C True
D True
E False

A single scan in the third trimester is of no value for clarifying the dates, or distinguishing wrong dates from a small baby. However, asymmetrical growth retardation due to placental insufficiency could be diagnosed as can anencephaly and fetal ascites. It is not yet possible to diagnose Down's syndrome by ultrasound.

212 Human chorionic gonadotrophin

A is secreted by the cytotrophoblast
B prevents degeneration of the corpus luteum
C is a good measure of placental function
D is secreted in maternal urine
E reaches maximum levels in the last trimester

213 The following are indications for performing a classical Caesarean section:

A breech presentation
B carcinoma of the cervix
C previous classical Caesarean section
D abruptio placentae
E severe fetal distress

214 An intra-uterine death can be managed by

A waiting for the spontaneous onset of labour
B artificial rupture of the membranes and oxytocin
C intra-amniotic prostaglandins
D extra-amniotic prostaglandins
E artificial rupture of the membranes alone

212 A True
    B True
    C False
    D True
    E False

Human chorionic gonadotrophin (HCG) is secreted by the inner cytotrophoblastic (Langhan's) layer of cells. Its presence in the maternal urine is used as the basis of most pregnancy tests and is maximal at about 60 days. It is no measure of placental function but is present in large amounts in trophoblastic disease (hydatidiform mole or choriocarcinoma) and is thus used for diagnosis and for monitoring response to treatment.

213 A False
    B True
    C False
    D False
    E False

The classical Caesarean section is a bad operation because of the considerable risk of scar rupture during the next labour or in late pregnancy. It should be performed however where there is a cervical carcinoma to keep the incision as far as possible from the lesion and of course it is justified for a rapid post-mortem Caesarean section. There is a trend towards delivering the very premature breech by Caesarean section at a time when the lower segment has yet to form. The improvement in perinatal health achieved by this considerable future risk to the mother has yet to be clarified.

214 A True
    B False
    C False
    D True
    E False

When a diagnosis of intra-uterine death has been made spontaneous labour can be awaited but this should not be for too long because of the risk of coagulation defects—and for obvious humanitarian reasons. The method of choice is to use prostaglandins extra-amniotically. The membranes should be left intact as long as possible because of the risk of intra-uterine infection, although with the effective use of oxytocin this is less of a danger.

215 Amniocentesis may be used for the diagnosis of
    A   sickle cell disease
    B   Tay–Sachs disease
    C   post-maturity
    D   microcephaly
    E   hydrops fetalis

216 The contractions of the uterus in pregnancy
    A   begin at the onset of labour
    B   are painless
    C   are reduced in intensity by orciprenaline
    D   increase in strength and frequency during labour
    E   are augmented with ergometrine

217 A pre-term fetus
    A   is born less than 37 completed weeks of gestation
    B   is born weighing less than 2.5 kg
    C   should be delivered by forceps
    D   has an increased risk of passing meconium in utero
    E   is at risk of developing hyaline membrane disease

218 The pain associated with uterine contractions may be relieved by the following methods:
    A   administration of diazepam
    B   intra-muscular pethidine
    C   pudendal block
    D   inhalation of entonox
    E   caudal block

215 A False
B True
C False
D False
E False

A genetic amniocentesis may be used to diagnose chromosomal abnormalities, sex-linked diseases and many of the inborn errors of metabolism such as Tay–Sachs disease. It can be used to assess rhesus disease but can not diagnose hydrops. Similarly many syndromes associated with mental defect or microcephaly may be diagnosed but microcephaly is at best a difficult ultrasonic diagnosis in the mid-trimester and is usually not diagnosed until after birth.

216 A False
B True
C True
D True
E False

Uterine contractions occur throughout pregnancy. The irregular painless contractions which occur before the onset of labour are called Braxton Hicks contractions. During labour these increase in frequency and strength. Contractions can be augmented by oxytocin but not by ergometrine which causes a prolonged tetanic contraction.

217 A True
B False
C False
D False
E True

The accepted definition of a pre-term infant is correctly given in (A). A baby may be born weighing less than 2.5 kg, but can be growth-retarded and not pre-term. The baby should be delivered carefully with control of the head and an episiotomy but forceps are not always necessary. The incidence of meconium-staining of the liquor increases as gestation progresses but is low in pre-term labours. The main risk facing a pre-term baby is hyaline membrane disease.

218 A False
B True
C False
D True
E True

Administration of diazepam will sedate but will not give analgesia. Pethidine and entonox on the other hand will provide some pain relief. A caudal block will relieve the pain of labour if it reaches spinal segments T11 and T12. A pudendal block will only provide analgesia to the perineum.

219 The station of the head in labour can be measured by
    A   the relationship to the ischial tuberosities
    B   the abdominal assessment
    C   its relationship to the ischial spines
    D   the amount of moulding which has occurred
    E   the degree of caput formation

220 The first stage of labour
    A   ends at full dilatation of the cervix
    B   begins when the membranes rupture
    C   can be shortened by the use of oxytocin
    D   normally lasts for more than 24 hr in primigravid women
    E   can be shortened by the use of obstetric forceps

221 The third stage of labour
    A   ends with the delivery of the placenta
    B   is shortened by the use of oxytocic drugs
    C   should not last longer than 5 min
    D   is prolonged with an epidural block
    E   begins as soon as the infant's head is delivered

222 Oxytocin
    A   is a steroid hormone
    B   has an anti-diuretic effect
    C   is produced in the anterior lobe of the pituitary gland
    D   may be used for the induction of labour
    E   is inactivated if swallowed

223 The complications of pregnancy in the diabetic patient include
    A   intra-uterine growth retardation
    B   polyhydramnios
    C   breech presentation
    D   increased risk of congenital malformation
    E   sudden intra-uterine death

219 A False
  B True
  C True
  D False
  E False

The level of the presenting head in labour is best assessed by establishing the number of fifths which remain above the pelvic brim. This can be done by abdominal or vaginal examination. The station can also be assessed on vaginal examination by assessing the relationship of the head to the ischial spines. This is measured in centimetres above or below the spines.

220 A True
  B False
  C True
  D False
  E False

The first stage of labour lasts from the onset of labour to full dilatation of the cervix. Although the onset may occasionally coincide with rupture of the membranes this is not normally the case. Labour usually lasts for less than 24 hr in primigravid patients and its duration can be reduced with an oxytocin infusion, although this should only be done if there are specific indications. Obstetric forceps should not be used before full dilatation of the cervix.

221 A True
  B True
  C False
  D False
  E False

The third stage of labour extends from the delivery of the baby until the completion of the delivery of the placenta. This may take up to 20 min but can be shortened by the use of oxytocic drugs and the active management of the third stage. The active management of the third stage also reduces the chance of haemorrhage.

222 A False
  B True
  C False
  D True
  E True

Oxytocin is secreted by the posterior pituitary and does have a weak anti-diuretic effect. This can be a problem when used in high concentrations for a prolonged period of time. It is used intravenously for the induction of labour but cannot be used orally. Buccal pitocin is no longer used.

223 A True
  B True
  C False
  D True
  E True

Most of the complications of diabetes in pregnancy are reduced if control is good. Congenital abnormalities are common if control is poor in early pregnancy and sudden fetal death if control is poor later in pregnancy. Intra-uterine growth retardation may occur if vascular changes are severe.

224 **An external cephalic version in the antenatal period is contra-indicated under the following circumstances:**
   A   polyhydramnios
   B   previous Caesarean section
   C   primigravid patients
   D   following ante-partum haemorrhage
   E   hypertension

225 **Beta sympathomimetic drugs should not be used**
   A   before 30 weeks
   B   with ruptured membranes
   C   if the estimated birth weight is more than 2.5 kg
   D   in the presence of pre-eclampsia
   E   with dexamethazone

226 **The pre-term fetus with a cephalic presentation should be delivered**
   A   usually by Caesarean section
   B   using a vacuum extractor
   C   by careful control of the head and an episiotomy
   D   with forceps
   E   in a caul

227 **The following drugs stop contractions:**
   A   alcohol
   B   magnesium sulphate
   C   corticosteroids
   D   salbutamol
   E   pethidine

224 A False
B True
C False
D True
E True

There is still argument as to whether external cephalic version should be used at all in obstetrics. It should not be performed where there is a Caesarean section scar because of the risk of a scar demiscence. If it is performed following an APH or when hypertension is present the risk of abruptio placentae is increased.

225 A False
B True
C True
D True
E False

Beta sympathomimetic drugs stop contractions but there is some debate whether they really prolong pregnancy. There is no debate about the dangers of these drugs and one should remember that 50% of patients in pre-term labour stop without any therapy. Tocolytic drugs should be reserved for pregnancies less than 34 weeks, babies weighing less than 2 kg with the membranes intact, the cervix closed, no hypertension, no APH, and no other major maternal or fetal complications. In these cases delivery might be advisable for both fetal and maternal indications.

226 A False
B False
C True
D False
E True

It is important to protect the head in a pre-term delivery. Traditionally forceps have been advised, but this might even be harmful. Certainly careful control with an episiotomy is to be preferred. Head protection is also achieved by delaying membrane rupture and if possible the premature fetus can be delivered with membranes intact (in a caul—like David Copperfield!).

227 A True
B True
C False
D True
E False

Beta sympathomimetic drugs are the most effective means of stopping contractions but should always be used with caution, for correct indications and in mothers without cardiac disease, hypertension or an ante-partum haemorrhage. Pethidine sedates but will not stop contractions. Corticosteroids are used to stimulate production of surfactant, and are often used in combination with tocolytic drugs.

228 The following names are associated with obstetric procedures
- **A** Schiller
- **B** Mauriceau
- **C** Lovset
- **D** Brandt Andrews
- **E** Fothergill

229 The following precautions should be taken before Caesarean section:
- **A** antacids should be given
- **B** pre-medication with pethidine and atropine should be given
- **C** the bladder should be catheterized
- **D** the patient should be lying flat on her back
- **E** signed consent for hysterectomy must be obtained

230 A transverse lie in labour
- **A** should be delivered by Caesarean section
- **B** should have a gentle attempt at internal podalic version
- **C** is caused by an abnormal uterus
- **D** is caused by an abnormal fetus
- **E** may be delivered by a destructive operation

231 The Dubowitz scoring system
- **A** is a method to assess the 'ripeness' of the cervix
- **B** is a method to assess the gestational age of a neonate
- **C** is a measure of fetal condition at birth
- **D** uses neurological criteria of maturity
- **E** predicts the presence of cephalo-pelvic disproportion

228 A False
B True
C True
D True
E False

The Schiller test is the application of iodine on the cervix to demonstrate glycogen negative areas and the Fothergill operation is the Manchester repair for uterine prolapse. The Mauriceau–Smellie–Veit manoeuvre is used to deliver the after-coming head of a breech and Lovset's manoeuvre is used to deliver extended arms. The Brandt Andrews method of controlled cord traction is the routine way of delivering the placenta after oxytocic administration.

229 A True
B False
C True
D False
E False

Pre-medication with atropine should be given but narcotics should be avoided as they depress the fetus. 10–15° of lateral tilt should be used to avoid supine hypotension. Although the risk of aspiration is small, with an experienced anaesthetist, an antacid should be given and cricoid pressure applied to reduce the chance of Mendelson's syndrome. It is good to be prepared but consent for hysterectomy is really going too far.

230 A True
B False
C True
D True
E True

If the fetus is alive, a transverse lie should be delivered by Caesarean section. This is also true if the fetus is dead unless the operator is extremely skilled in destructive procedures, such as decapitation using a Blond–Heidler saw if the cervix is fully dilated. Internal podalic version should never be used in view of the risk of uterine rupture unless transverse lie occurs in a second twin with intact membranes.

231 A False
B True
C False
D True
E False

The gestational age of a neonate may be assessed by using the Dubowitz scoring system which combines neurological and physical criteria of maturity. It is particularly useful when deciding whether a low birthweight infant is pre-term or growth retarded. The 'ripeness' of the cervix is assessed by the Bishop score, fetal condition at birth is assessed by the Agpar score and cephalo-pelvic disproportion is in most cases only diagnosed by a trial of labour.

232 Secondary post-partum haemorrhage
- **A** occurs more than 24 hr after delivery
- **B** is often associated with intra-uterine infection
- **C** is reduced by the active management of the third stage of labour
- **D** should be treated with ergometrine
- **E** usually needs a currettage

233 Maternal rubella infection in early pregnancy
- **A** causes blindness in the infant
- **B** leads to hydrocephaly in the infant
- **C** can be diagnosed by a single high antibody titre
- **D** commonly results in spontaneous abortion
- **E** causes thrombocytopenic purpura in the infant

234 The Apgar score of the neonate takes into consideration the
- **A** heart rate
- **B** colour of the skin
- **C** moro reflex
- **D** respiratory rate
- **E** muscle tone

235 The Dubowitz score of the neonate
- **A** is assessed immediately after delivery
- **B** is scored out of ten
- **C** includes physical features
- **D** includes neurological features
- **E** assess the time length of amenorrhoea

232 A True
B True
C False
D False
E True

Secondary post-partum haemorrhage (sometimes called puerperal haemorrhage) occurs following the first 24 hr after delivery and is most commonly associated with retained products of conception, particularly membranes and retained blood clot and also infection. Ergometrine is not helpful. Antibiotics are often indicated and evacuation of uterus is usually required. This evacuation should be done extremely carefully as the uterus is very easily perforated soon after delivery.

233 A True
B True
C True
D False
E True

Rubella was first described in Australia in 1941 as a major cause of fetal abnormality, causing cardiac lesion, cataracts, deafness, mental retardation, hepatosplenomegaly and thrombocytopenic purpura. The maternal disease is not severe and does not predispose to miscarriage. It can be diagnosed by a single raised IgM titre, but two or three rising levels of IgG would be required. If active infection in the first trimester is confirmed, termination of pregnancy is indicated.

234 A True
B True
C False
D False
E True

The Apgar score is used to assess neonatal condition at 1 and 5 min of life. Heart rate, respiratory rhythm, skin colour, muscle tone and response to stimulation are assessed. There is a good correlation between 5-min Apgar score and subsequent infant development.

235 A False
B False
C True
D True
E False

The Dubowitz score is used to assess neonatal gestational age which may not be related to period of amenorrhoea. It involves a fairly complex assessment of physical external characteristics and neurological features. The maximum score is 70.

236 Gas shadows in the great vessels of the fetus on radiological examination are associated with
A duodenal atresia
B amniotic fluid infection syndrome
C anencephaly
D intra-uterine death
E exomphalos

237 Glucose 6 phosphate dehydrogenase deficiency (G6PD)
A is a cause of anaemia in pregnancy
B is associated with drug-induced haemolysis
C is associated with neonatal jaundice
D is confirmed by haemoglobin electrophoresis
E is sex-linked

238 X-ray pelvimetry may be performed for the following indications:
A brow presentation in labour
B a previous Caesarean section
C high head at term
D primigravid breech presentation
E transverse lie at term

239 Signs of placental separation are
A the fundus of the uterus relaxes
B there is a small 'gush' of blood
C the cord lengthens
D abolished by the use of ergometrine
E the fundus of the uterus rises

236 A False
B False
C False
D True
E False

Gas can only form in the fetal blood vessels after intra-uterine death. The bubbles seen on ultra-sound examination in cases of intestinal malformation are fluid filled bubbles. Amniotic fluid infection syndrome may rarely be due to gas forming organisms but the gas is not inside the fetus.

237 A False
B True
C True
D False
E True

G6PD is a disease found in patients originating from Africa, the Mediterranean, the Middle and Far East. Drug-induced jaundice and neonatal jaundice are important features. It is sex-linked, occurring only in males, and is confirmed by testing the enzyme activity of red cells: this should be performed after birth in areas of increased incidence (e.g. S.E. Asia).

238 A False
B True
C False
D True
E False

Radiology can provide a very accurate assessment of the pelvic dimensions and is particularly useful when assessing the mode of delivery in breech presentations and where there has been one previous Caesarean section for a non-recurring cause. It is pointless to perform pelvimetry when the mode of delivery will be Caesarean section regardless of the pelvic dimensions.

239 A False
B True
C True
D False
E True

The signs of placental separation should be awaited before the placenta is actively delivered and on no account should controlled cord traction be employed before the uterus has contracted. In fact only lengthening of the cord is a good sign of placental separation as the traditional gush of blood and rising uterine fundus also indicates a post-partum haemorrhage. Nevertheless, they are text-book signs of placental separation.

240 Pregnancy-induced hypertension is associated with
A a blood pressure rise in the first trimester of pregnancy
B proteinuria
C abnormal liver function
D hypertension which persists
E intra-vascular coagulation

241 The following factors predisposed to pregnancy-induced hypertension (pre-eclampsia):
A multiple pregnancy
B multigravidity
C hydatidiform mole
D chronic renal disease
E anaemia

242 The following management should be instituted in a patient found to have moderate pregnancy-induced hypertension at the antenatal clinic:
A admission to hospital for bed rest
B commence an oral hypotensive agent
C commence diazepam
D commence a diuretic
E monitor fetal growth

243 Malaria in pregnancy
A causes fetal abnormalities
B cause pre-term labour
C should be treated with chloroquine
D causes intra-uterine growth retardation
E is diagnosed by culture of the organism

240 A False
 B True
 C True
 D False
 E True

The rise in blood pressure in pregnancy-induced hypertension (pre-eclampsia) usually occurs in the second half of pregnancy. Proteinuria is a sign of severe disease. Hepatic changes are common and disseminated intra-vascular coagulation is an essential feature of the disease, although it is certainly not causative.

241 A True
 B False
 C True
 D False
 E False

Pregnancy-induced hypertension is by definition hypertension occurring with or without proteinuria in patients without renal or cardiovascular disease. The aetiology remains unknown but certain predisposing factors can be identified. These are primigravidity, early age of pregnancy, multiple pregnancy, hydatidiform mole, the presence of hydrops fetalis and of course the overwhelming effect of socio and nutritional deprivation.

242 A True
 B False
 C False
 D False
 E True

The most important feature in the management of pregnancy-induced hypertension is bed rest. Oral hypotensive agents may have a place in early pregnancy but not until the response of the blood pressure to bed rest has been assessed. Diazepam should not be used as long-term treatment and diuretics should also be avoided. Fetal growth and health should be monitored carefully by whatever means are available. Fetal movements are extremely useful, possibly the best and certainly the cheapest test of fetal wellbeing.

243 A False
 B True
 C True
 D True
 E False

Malaria in pregnancy is common in many developing countries. It may cause abortion, pre-term labour, growth retardation but not congenital abnormalities. Attacks can be prevented with prophylactic chloroquine or other anti-malarials. The diagnosis is made by staining blood smears for parasites and the first line treatment is a full course of chloroquine.

244 Eclampsia is successfully treated by
- **A** intra-muscular diazepam
- **B** chlormethiazole
- **C** calcium gluconate
- **D** magnesium sulphate
- **E** hydrallazine

245 The following drugs should never be used in pregnancy
- **A** progestogens
- **B** diazepam
- **C** tetracycline
- **D** diethylstilboestrol
- **E** propranolol

246 Fetal lung maturity may be assessed by
- **A** X-rays
- **B** the L/S ratio
- **C** the shake test
- **D** the Nile blue-staining technique
- **E** measuring the amount of lecithin in the liquor

244 A False
B True
C False
D True
E False

There are many methods which have been used to control the convulsions in eclampsia. It is important for any obstetric unit to choose one of these methods and not to indulge in polypharmacy. Effective methods are intravenous diazepam, chlormethiazole and magnesium sulphate. Intramuscular diazepam is not effective. Calcium gluconate is used to remove the respiratory depression which may occur with magnesium sulphate. Hydrallazine is a hypotensive agent.

245 A True
B False
C True
D True
E False

Masculinization of the female fetus has been noted after maternal treatment with progestogens and DES may cause clear cell adenocarcinoma of the vagina in the children of mothers treated in early pregnancy. Tetracycline causes permanent staining of deciduous teeth and irreversible depression of bone growth. Diazepam should not be used for long-term ante-partum therapy but may be used intravenously for the acute management of severe pre-eclampsia. Propranolol may be useful in cardiac disease, but should be avoided if possible as it crosses the placenta and can cause prolonged adrenergic blockade.

246 A False
B True
C True
D False
E True

The most important factor associated with lung function maturity is the amount of lecithin in the liquor. This can be measured directly, or indirectly by means of the L/S ratio or the shake test. The Nile blue-staining technique is a method to assess skin maturity by assessing the percentage of fat containing cells in desquamated fetal cells.

247 Reliable and safe methods of placental localization are

A soft tissue radiography
B anteriography
C radio isotope placentography
D thermography
E ultrasound

248 A patient with tight mitral stenosis in pregnancy

A should receive prophylactic antibiotics in labour
B should be delivered by Caesarean section
C may sometimes have a mitral valvotomy performed
D should be given intravenous ergometrine in the third stage
E should have adequate analgesia in labour

249 An intra-uterine death may be confirmed by

A a positive Spalding's sign
B ultrasound
C the presence of gas in the amniotic fluid
D serum oestrogen levels
E urinary HCG levels

250 Cholestatic jaundice of pregnancy

A has a high incidence among Scandinavians
B is associated with pruritus
C does not lead to chronic liver disease
D is associated with recurrence if oral oestrogen-containing contraceptives are used
E is an indication for termination of pregnancy

247 A False
  B False
  C False
  D False
  E True

The standard method for localizing the placenta is now ultrasound. Radio isotope placentography and thermography do not give a satisfactory degree of accuracy and reliability and arteriography although accurate is associated with too many maternal complications. In spite of ultrasonography it may still be necessary to ultimately diagnose the position of the placenta by an examination under anaesthesia in theatre.

248 A True
  B False
  C True
  D False
  E True

If there is rapid deterioration in the condition of a patient with mitral stenosis in pregnancy, mitral valvotomy may be considered but it is rarely performed. In the absence of other problems the patient should be allowed to labour but prophylactic antibiotics should be used together with adequate analgesia. Intravenous ergometrine should not be used as this increases the venous return to the heart.

249 A True
  B True
  C False
  D False
  E False

An intra-uterine death is best diagnosed by ultrasound in the absence of fetal heart or fetal movement, however in many parts of the world X-ray diagnosis with the traditional radiological signs will be the best available method. These signs are overlapping of the skull bones (Spalding sign), gas in the great vessels (Robert's sign), a halo appearance of the scalp and a crumpled hyperflexed appearance of the fetal spine.

250 A True
  B True
  C True
  D True
  E False

Intra-hepatic cholestasis in pregnancy is uncommon but has a higher incidence in some regions —for example in Scandinavia. In general, pruritus is usually a feature and precedes the onset of jaundice. The prognosis is good but the patient should be advised not to use oestrogen-containing contraceptives in the future as this may cause a recurrence.

251 **Superficial thrombophlebitis in the puerperium**
   A   occurs in about 5% of pregnancies
   B   predisposes to pulmonary embolism
   C   is treated with rest and local support
   D   should be treated with antibiotics
   E   is associated with an elevation in temperature

252 **Asymptomatic bacteriuria occurs**
   A   in 2% of pregnant women
   B   is associated with an increased perinatal mortality
   C   predisposes to acute pyelonephritis
   D   is defined as a bacterial count in excess of 10,000 organisms/ml
   E   should be checked at each antenatal visit

253 **Chronic renal disease in pregnancy is associated with an increased incidence of**
   A   premature labour
   B   placenta praevia
   C   accidental haemorrhage
   D   anaemia
   E   asymmetric growth retardation

254 **The progress of labour may be assessed by**
   A   measurement of the strength of contraction
   B   assessment of cervical dilatation every 4 hr
   C   auscultation of the fetal heart rate
   D   assessment of the descent of the head
   E   measurement of the amount of caput formation

251 A False
    B False
    C True
    D False
    E True

Superficial thrombophlebitis occurs in about 1% of pregnancies. Unlike deep vein thrombosis it does not lead to pulmonary embolism. The inflammation is not due to infection and chemotherapy is not necessary. Local support and rest however can be helpful. Although the temperature may be elevated, this is usually only mild.

252 A False
    B True
    C True
    D False
    E False

Asymptomatic bacteria has a culture of 100,000 or more organisms per ml and should be checked at the booking visit. It occurs in approximately 5% of pregnancies and is associated with chronic renal abnormalities, acute pyelonephritis in 25% of affected patients and has a slightly increased perinatal mortality in view of the increased frequency of hypertension in patients with chronic renal disease. It is usual to treat this condition with a single course of ampicillin.

253 A True
    B False
    C True
    D True
    E True

Normotensive chronic renal disease has an excellent prognosis in pregnancy as the principle prognostic feature is a degree of hypertension followed by a degree impairment of renal function. Hypertension may produce abruption, fetal growth retardation, prematurity, fetal distress and an increased incidence of intra-uterine growth retardation.

254 A False
    B True
    C False
    D True
    E False

The only precise arbiters of the progress of labour are the dilatation of cervix and descent of the presenting part. Assessment of fetal heart characteristics is for the diagnosis of fetal distress. Caput formation indicates a difficult or prolonged labour. Assessment of strength of contractions either by palpition, intrauterine monitoring or the amount of pain present tells us nothing about the efficiency of first stage progress.

255 Induction of labour may be achieved by
A artificial rupture of the membranes
B intravenous infusion of alcohol
C extra amniotic prostaglandin E2
D beta sympathomomimetic drugs
E indomethacin suppositories

256 The prolonged latent phase:
A characteristically occurs after unwise induction of labour
B is usually followed by a slow active phase
C is due to cephalo-pelvic disproportion
D is associated with premature membrane rupture
E is appropriately treated by sedation

257 Primary dysfunctional labour is caused by:
A cephalo-pelvic disproportion
B dysfunctional uterine action
C occipito-posterior position
D fetal distress
E lumbar epidural block

258 The complications of amniocentesis in late pregnancy include
A premature membrane rupture
B chorio-amnionitis
C rhesus immunization
D spina bifida
E bowel perforation

255 A True
 B False
 C True
 D False
 E False

Labour may be induced by rupturing the fore-waters artificially or by the insertion of intra-vaginal or extra amniotic prostaglandins E2 or F2 alpha. The other answers are all method of stopping labour although only the beta sympathomomimetic drugs ritodrine or salbutamol are really used today. Alcohol makes a patient feel ill and indomethacin, a prostaglandin inhibitor, can cause premature closure of the ductus arteriosus.

256 A True
 B False
 C False
 D True
 E True

A prolonged latent phase is one of the three aberrant cervimetric patterns of the first stage, the other two being dysfunctional labour and second-ary arrest. It is characteristically due to induction of labour, premature membrane rupture or heavy sedation very early in labour and is not due to disproportion. Although believed to be a fairly benign abnormality it does carry a Caesarean sec-tion rate of almost 20% and the management is controversial. However, sedation and oxytocin are acceptable means of treatment.

257 A True
 B True
 C True
 D False
 E False

Primary dysfunctional labour is defined as a first stage when progress in the active phase is less than 1 cm/hr. It is typically due to disproportion, poor contractions, deflection of the head or an occipito posterior position. It should be treated with augmentation by oxytocin and with careful fetal monitoring and good pain relief. An epidural block does not alter the progress of the first stage.

258 A True
 B True
 C True
 D False
 E False

Amniocentesis can be valuable in late pregnancy in order to measure the L/S ratio and assess fetal lung maturity. The placenta should be localized before the procedure by ultrasound in order to reduce the risk of feto-maternal transfusion and immunization of a rhesus negative mother. Chorio-amnionitis is very rare as the amniotic fluid is bactericidal but it may occur and full sterile precautions should be taken.

259 Spina Bifida
- **A** is more common in Africa than U.K.
- **B** is characteristically diagnosed by a high amniotic fluid placental lactogen
- **C** is diagnosed by ultrasound at 18 weeks
- **D** is due to autosomal recessive gene
- **E** is associated with polyhydramnios

260 Separation of the symphysis pubis
- **A** occurs during the antenatal period
- **B** is accompanied by a high fever
- **C** causes tenderness over the symphysis
- **D** is detected by 'springing' the pelvis
- **E** is managed by surgery

261 A craniotomy is appropriate treatment in developing countries
- **A** when the fetus is hydrocephalic
- **B** in obstructed labour with fetal distress
- **C** for a transverse lie with a prolapse arm
- **D** where the fetus is anencephalic
- **E** in obstructed labour at full dilatation with a dead fetus

259 A False
B False
C True
D False
E True

Spina bifida is 'the curse of the Celts' occurring much more commonly in the U.K. than anywhere else in the world. It can be diagnosed by alpha-fetoprotein assays when the lesion is open. Closed spina bifidas are more difficult to recognize but ultrasound is now a more precise means of diagnosis. There is no recognizable chromosomal abnormality associated with neural tube defect. Spina bifidas produce polyhydramnios presumably due to transfer of fluid and CSF through the sac membranes.

260 A True
B False
C True
D True
E False

Separation of the symphysis pubis may occur at any time during pregnancy although it most commonly presents after delivery. The characteristic signs are tenderness above the symphysis and palpition and on applying pressure to both iliac crests simultaneously (springing test). The management of the condition is conservative with bed rest, analgesics and physiotherapy. If tenderness over the symphysis is accompanied by a severe febrile illness osteitis pubis should be suspected.

261 A True
B False
C False
D False
E True

In developed countries craniotomy is now a rare operation except for the delivery of a hydrocephalic fetus which presents as an obstructed labour. In developing countries where obstructed labour is more common it may be used to deliver a dead fetus, but only if the cervix is fully dilated and the head is presenting. In this way the patient will be spared a uterine scar which might be a lethal complication.

262 Anencephalic fetus is associated with
- **A** post-maturity
- **B** oligohydramnios
- **C** high maternal oestriol levels
- **D** increased incidence of Caesarean section
- **E** shoulder dystocia

263 Artificial rupture of the membranes
- **A** should be performed under general anaesthetic or epidural block
- **B** should not be performed until the patient is approaching full dilatation
- **C** is used to induce labour
- **D** should be accompanied by 'sweeping' the membranes
- **E** is more efficient if the hind waters are ruptured

264 In the active phase of labour
- **A** an epidural block slows progress
- **B** the cervix dilates at a rate of more than 1 cm/min
- **C** the fetal head should be engaged
- **D** oxytocin cannot be used
- **E** the membranes should be ruptured

262 **A** True
B False
C False
D False
E True

Anencephalics should now be diagnosed in the first trimester by alpha-fetoprotein screening or by ultrasound. The fetal pituitary gland is poorly developed hence there is no ACTH to stimulate the fetal adrenal. This may cause failure to start labour at term and extreme post-maturity. There is however a more frequent association with poly-hydramnios and premature labour. Dystocia in labour may occur if the small head slips through an incompletely dilated cervix and also shoulder dystocia may occur.

263 **A** False
B False
C True
D False
E False

Artificial rupture of the membranes is usually performed as a low amniotomy in the active phase of labour in order to stimulate contractions, to observe the colour of the amniotic fluid and to apply a scalp electrode. It can also be used alone or in conjunction with oxytocic drugs in order to induce labour. Once the membranes are ruptured the risk of ascending infection is increased particularly if a membrane 'sweep' is also performed.

264 **A** False
B True
C False
D False
E True

The active phase follows the latent phase, begins at approximately 3 cm and proceeds at a rate in excess of 1 cm/min. If the progress of the first stage is slower than this, oxytocin should be used to accelerate labour. It is advisable to rupture the membranes in the active phase. This aids contractions, facilitates the use of a scalp electrode and enables meconium-stained amniotic fluid to be identified. Epidural analgesia often has a profound effect upon the second stage but does not alter the progress of the first stage.

265 A vacuum extractor (Ventouse) may be used to assist delivery for
A   pre-term delivery
B   an occipito posterior position of the head
C   delay in the second stage where the head is three-fifths above the pelvic brim
D   fetal distress at full dilatation
E   the after-coming head

266 The following maternal infections may damage the fetus:
A   viral hepatitis
B   rubella
C   herpes
D   cytomegalovirus
E   toxoplasmosis

267 Prostaglandins are:
A   synthesized from cholesterol
B   secreted by the pituitary gland
C   secreted by the prostate gland
D   oxytocic
E   associated with gastro-intestinal side effects

268 Multiple pregnancies
A   may be diagnosed at 8 weeks' gestation by ultrasound
B   occur in about 1 in 80 pregnancies in caucasian patients
C   are more common with increased maternal age
D   should not be allowed to proceed beyond 38 weeks' gestation
E   should have bed rest for approximately 4 weeks in late pregnancy

265 **A** False
B True
C False
D True
E False

Vacuum extraction is a useful technique which must also be used with great care. Only three pulls are allowed with good maternal effort throughout three entire contractions. It is ideal for the occipito posterior position or the deep transverse arrest in a tight funnel pelvis in the presence of moulding. It may be used with the head two-fifths above the brim, but the head will not come down—safely—if it is three or more fifths above the brim.

266 **A** True
B True
C True
D True
E True

Any systemic infection especially in early pregnancy may damage the fetus. Currently interest centres on the TORCH group (toxoplasmosis, rubella, cytomegalovirus and herpes). They are associated with spontaneous abortion, fetal abnormalities, hydrops fetalis and intra-uterine death. Blood antibodies and immunoglobulins may aid diagnosis.

267 **A** False
B False
C True
D True
E True

Prostaglandins, originally isolated from male prostatic secretions, have since been isolated from many body fluids. They are synthesized from arachidonic acid, are not steroids and are not pituitary hormones. Their most important effects are on the female reproductive tract. Their systemic use is limited by gastro-intestinal side-effects.

268 **A** True
B True
C True
D False
E False

Multiple pregnancy occurs in about 1 in 80 in caucasians, more commonly in negroid races and less commonly in far eastern races. It can be diagnosed by ultrasound in early pregnancy or by X-ray after the twentieth week. They present many obstetric complications particularly prematurity, but neither bed rest nor a cervical cerclage improves the prognosis.

269 The following are associated with Down's syndrome:
- **A** trisomy 15
- **B** balanced translocation
- **C** congenital heart disease
- **D** diagnosis by ultrasound
- **E** increased incidence with increasing maternal age

270 Deep vein thrombosis in pregnancy
- **A** is more common in older women
- **B** is often asymptomatic
- **C** should be treated with intravenous heparin
- **D** should be treated with warfarin towards term
- **E** needs investigation by venography

271 The after-coming head of a breech is safely delivered by
- **A** supra-pubic pressure
- **B** forceps
- **C** the Burns–Marshall technique
- **D** Lovset's manoeuvre
- **E** Mauriceau–Smellie–Veit manoeuvre

272 Epidural analgesia
- **A** can be achieved by the lumbar or caudal route
- **B** is associated with hypotension
- **C** is associated prolonged severe backache
- **D** should not be used in the presence of severe haemorrhage
- **E** should not be used in pre-term labour

269 A False
    B True
    C True
    D False
    E True

Down's syndrome is trisomy 21 which will occur in 1% of pregnancies at the age of 40 and 5% in pregnancies age 44. There is also a less dramatic increased incidence with paternal age from the age of 50. It is usually diagnosed by amniocentesis and culture of fetal cells. Its features are a characteristic facies with slanting eyes and epicanthic folds, short hands with abnormal skin creases, mental deficiency and congenital heart disease.

270 A False
    B True
    C True
    D False
    E True

Deep vein thrombosis is a serious complication which may lead to pulmonary embolism. It now complicates the antenatal period as frequently as the puerperium. The classical signs and symptoms are absent in over 50% of patients and venography is often necessary to confirm the diagnosis and to recognize any ascending ileo-femoral extension. Heparin is the usual treatment followed by warfarin which should be avoided in the first trimester and in the last few weeks of pregnancy.

271 A False
    B True
    C True
    D False
    E True

The most important aspect of the delivery of the head of a breech is careful control and forceps to the after-coming head is the best way to achieve this. However, the Mauriceau–Smellie–Veit method of head flexion and traction is acceptable and the Burns–Marshall is traditional but probably less good. Lovset's manoeuvre is used for the delivery of extended arms.

272 A True
    B True
    C False
    D True
    E False

Epidural analgesia is an excellent means of pain relief which can be achieved by either the lumbar or the caudal epidural spaces. The lumbar route is generally preferred at the level of L3-L4 or L4-L5. Hypotension can be prevented by pre-loading the circulation with fluid. A severe headache is common when a dural tap occurs. Backache is not a feature. The relaxation obtained is ideal for use with pre-term labour, a breech or twins.

273 **The 'ripeness' of the cervix**
  A   is assessed by Bishop score
  B   is improved by oxytocin infusion
  C   is improved by intra-vaginal prostaglandins
  D   is influenced by the head level
  E   bears a relationship to the need for augmentation of labour

274 **The following maternal diseases are usually aggravated by pregnancy**
  A   gastric ulcer
  B   hiatus hernia
  C   diabetes
  D   multiple sclerosis
  E   rheumatoid arthritis

275 **The following are associated with rupture of a Caesarean section scar in labour:**
  A   slow progress of labour
  B   fetal distress
  C   maternal tachycardia
  D   loss of bright red blood at the end of the first stage
  E   marked tenderness of the lower uterus

273 A True   The Bishop score assesses the pelvic factors in-
    B False   dicating the ripeness or the inducability of the
    C True   cervix. The factors considered are dilatation,
    D True   length, consistency and position of the cervix and
    E False   the head level. It has a numerical value up to 13
which predicts the ease of induction of labour (not
augmentation as this refers to acceleration of spontaneous labour). If the cervix is unfavourable (with
a Bishop score less than 5) it can be ripened with
intra-vaginal prostaglandins, but intravenous oxytocin is not useful.

274 A False   Gastric ulcer is rarely associated with pregnancy
    B True   but tends to improve because of the lower acid
    C True   secretion and motility, and increase in mucus pro-
    D True   duction. Hiatus hernia tends to be aggravated. The
    E False   endocrine and metabolic effects of pregnancy
usually aggravate diabetes with the insulin
requirement increasing. Multiple sclerosis also
tends to be aggravated in pregnancy but rheumatoid
arthritis often improves.

275 A False   In a patient who is labouring following a previous
    B True   Caesarean section, it is important to identify early
    C True   signs of impending rupture of the scar such as
    D True   tenderness over the scar, vaginal bleeding, fetal
    E True   tachycardia with maternal tachycardia occurring
later. Marked fetal distress is also a later sign with
disappearance of the fetal heart and contractions
when the uterus has ruptured. A classical scar is
more treacherous in that it tends to rupture before
labour starts and without any warning symptoms or
signs.

276 A primigravid patient whose cervix has been fully dilated for 30 min, with the head three-fifths above the pelvic brim, with caput and moulding, can be safely delivered by
  A lower segment Caesarean section
  B vacuum extraction
  C symphysiotomy and vacuum extraction
  D forceps delivery
  E internal version and breech extraction

277 The following are important in lactation
  A decreased progesterone
  B increased oestrogen
  C prolactin-releasing factor from the hypothalmus
  D formation of colostrum
  E oxytocin stimulation

278 The following complications are more common in association with a uterine abnormality:
  A placenta praevia
  B transverse lie
  C multiple pregnancy
  D acute pyelonephritis
  E ectopic pregnancy

276 A True
 B False
 C True
 D False
 E False

Head level is best described as 'fifths' of head above the brim. In this case the head is not engaged although the caput and moulding could bring the scalp to the vulva. The best method for delivery would be a Caesarean section. The head is too high to permit delivery by forceps or vacuum extraction. However, in certain circumstances in the Third World such a case with prolonged obstructed labour with intra-uterine infection might be best delivered by an experienced obstetrician using symphysiotomy followed by a vacuum extraction.

277 A False
 B False
 C False
 D False
 E True

The fall in oestrogen levels after delivery causes a reduction in prolactin-inhibiting factor from the hypothalmus. This leads to the release of prolactin from the anterior pituitary and the production of breast milk is initiated. Oxytocin is released from the posterior pituitary in response to suckling. It causes contractions of the myoepithelial cells, forcing milk into the lactiferous ducts.

278 A False
 B True
 C False
 D True
 E True

Uterine abnormality predisposes to malpresentation such as transverse lie, breech presentation and prolapsed arm in labour. A rudimentary horn may be the site of an ectopic pregnancy. As there is a frequent co-existent renal tract abnormality acute pyelonephritis is more common. Other problems include recurrent abortion or premature labour, ante-partum and post-partum haemorrhage and retained placenta.

279 Valid indications for induction of labour include
- **A** breech at 38 weeks
- **B** grand multiparity
- **C** previous Caesarean section
- **D** uncertain gestation
- **E** borderline cephalo-pelvic disproportion

280 A face presentation
- **A** occurs about one in every 2000 deliveries
- **B** is usually delivered by Caesarean section
- **C** presents the mento vertical diameter
- **D** is associated with hydrocephaly
- **E** most commonly presents as mento posterior

281 Internal podalic version may be performed for
- **A** breech presentation
- **B** obstructed brow presentation
- **C** first twin if transverse lie
- **D** second twin if transverse lie and membranes intact
- **E** intra-uterine death at full dilatation

279 A False
  B False
  C False
  D False
  E False

Induction of labour should be performed only for good indications as a Caesarean section will be necessary for a failed induction. The risks of induction are increased in grand multigravid patients and also in patients who had a previous Caesarean section. There is no reason to induce a breech at 38 weeks and induction is seriously contra-indicated if the head is high or there is any doubt about the size of the pelvis. A successful induction is more likely if the indications are valid and the Bishop (cervical) score is high.

280 A False
  B False
  C False
  D False
  E False

A face presentation occurs about once in every 300 deliveries. The most common position is with the chin pointing anteriorly (mento anterior) and in this position the baby can be delivered vaginally often with the aid of forceps. The presenting diameter is submento bregmatic and is 9.5 cm. Certain fetal abnormalities such as thyroid tumours or anencephaly predisposed to a face presentation.

281 A False
  B False
  C False
  D True
  E False

Internal podalic version is a procedure which should only be used at full dilatation with the membranes intact or having just ruptured with the uterus relaxing between contractions. These criteria only apply for a second twin. The risk of ruptured uterus when used for other indications given is too great to justify its use in these circumstances even in the harsh obstetric realities of the Third World.

282 Moulding of the fetal skull

- **A** is common where there is a posterior position of the occiput
- **B** can be measured using a moulding 'score'
- **C** disappears within 24 hr of delivery
- **D** leads to intra-cranial haemorrhage
- **E** is rare in pre-term infants

283 Convulsions after delivery may be due to

- **A** eclampsia
- **B** malaria
- **C** hypothyroidism
- **D** hypoglycaemia
- **E** idiopathic epilepsy

284 Abruptio placentae

- **A** is commoner in primigravid patients than multigravid patients
- **B** is associated with a 'Couvelaire' uterus
- **C** always causes vaginal bleeding
- **D** can lead to fetal death
- **E** is associated with cardiac disease

282 **A** True
B True
C True
D False
E False

Moulding is due to compression of the fetal skull as it passes through the pelvis. The head moulds more readily in the pre-term fetus although it can occur in the relatively hard or inelastic skull of the post-term baby. It is helpful to assess the degree of moulding using a moulding score as outlined below:

bones just touching $+$

bones overlapping but can be reduced $++$

bones overlapping but cannot be reduced $+++$

The moulding is assessed in relation to the sutures between the occipital and parietal bones plus both parietal bones. This gives a maximum possible score of $6+$.

283 **A** True
B True
C False
D True
E True

If post-partum convulsions are associated with hypertension and proteinuria the most likely diagnosis is eclampsia. Post-partum eclampsia is now more common than antenatal eclampsia in the U.K. probably due to the use of ergometrine in hypertensive patients for the third stage, and also due to improved antenatal care. It is also important to exclude other causes. Idiopathic epilepsy may be associated with transient proteinuria. Cerebral malaria and hypoglycaemia may present with coma, but can cause convulsions.

284 **A** False
B True
C False
D True
E False

Abruptio placentae (previously called accidental haemorrhage) is seen most commonly in multigravid patients. It is associated with hypertension, trauma or a rapid reduction in size of the uterus as it follows the release of polyhydramnios. In the majority of cases however no predisposing factor can be identified. The bleeding may be entirely concealed and it is especially in this situation that fetal death occurs. The blood may extravasate between muscle fibres to give the typical plum-coloured appearance of the 'Couvelaire' uterus.

285 **Sickle cell disease in pregnancy**
  A   is commoner in South Africa than in West Africa
  B   is associated with acute abdominal pain
  C   is a common cause of maternal death
  D   should be treated with repeated blood transfusion
  E   includes genotype SC

286 **A trial of labour**
  A   is usually induced
  B   can diagnose cephalopelvic disproportion
  C   should not have oxytocin stimulation
  D   is used in breech presentations
  E   should not be initiated if the head is not engaged

287 **The following conditions are more common in multiparous patients than primigravid patients**
  A   pre-eclampsia
  B   malpresentation
  C   post-partum haemorrhage
  D   anaemia
  E   prolonged labour

285
A False
B True
C True
D True
E True

It is amazing that sickle cell disease in pregnancy, a problem that was only first described in 1941, has now become the major cause of maternal death in parts of London. Sickle cell disease may be of genotype SS, SC or S.Thal. The main complications in pregnancy are anaemia, sickle cell crisis with bone pain and abdominal pain or infarction of the spleen or bone. Both perinatal mortality and maternal mortality are increased in patients with sickle cell disease, particularly where appropriate prophylactic measures have been omitted during pregnancy. These measures include folic acid, anti-malarials if appropriate and top up blood transfusions of normal blood if possible.

286
A False
B True
C False
D False
E False

A trial of labour is a well-conducted labour in a patient with a suspected small pelvis to see if good contractions will bring about flexion, a safe degree of moulding, descent and the vaginal delivery of a healthy baby. Ideally there should be spontaneous onset of labour. It is relevant to a cephalic presentation but never to a breech and by definition a trial of labour will occur frequently in patients where the head is not engaged.

287
A False
B True
C True
D True
E False

Multiparous patients may have more chronic hypertension but pre-eclampsia is not a problem. Similarly, although subsequent babies are often larger and unexpected obstructed labour is a treacherous problem in multigravid patients, prolonged labour is not more common. The poor third stage retraction may pre-dispose to an atonic form of post-partum haemorrhage.

288 **The following are indications for Caesarean section where the fetus is presenting by the breech:**
   A   meconium-stained amniotic fluid
   B   estimated weight of baby greater than 3.5 kg
   C   slow progress in the first stage of labour
   D   grand multiparous patients
   E   labour before 34 weeks

289 **Epidural analgesia in labour is contra-indicated in**
   A   cardiac disease
   B   multiple pregnancy
   C   severe ante-partum haemorrhage
   D   hypertension
   E   borderline cephalopelvic disproportion

290 **Fetal hypoxia should be managed by**
   A   maternal infusion of glucose
   B   delivery of the fetus
   C   observing the mother in the supine position
   D   maternal infusion of bicarbonate
   E   maternal sedation

288
A False
B True
C True
D False
E True

The causes of fetal mortality (in the Developed World) for breech presentation are fetal abnormality, cerebral haemorrhage and hypoxia—in that order. If there is any suggestion of disproportion such as estimated weight greater than 3.5 kg or slow first stage progress, the baby should be delivered by Caesarean section. Similarly the small breech of less than 1.5 kg whether it is premature or small for dates is probably better delivered by the abdominal route. Meconium-stained liquor is very common in breech presentation and should not, by itself, be taken as a sign of fetal distress.

289
A False
B False
C True
D False
E False

Epidural analgesia is an excellent means of pain relief but should not be used in the presence of severe haemorrhage. It is ideal for patients with hypertension as it may produce a slight decrease in the blood pressure. It may allow gentle pain-free manipulation necessary for twins or a breech delivery and is useful in borderline cephalopelvic disproportion as the pains of augmentation may be severe. If these patients come to a Caesarean section it is advisable to use the successful epidural block as the anaesthetic.

290
A False
B True
C False
D False
E False

If the fetus has been proved to be hypoxic because of fetal heart rate changes particularly loss of beat-to-beat variation or decelerations or bradycardia the best management is to deliver the baby as soon as possible. In the meantime the patient should be lying on her side and given oxygen by mask. Infusion of glucose and bicarbonate are not helpful.

291 Coagulation defects in pregnancy occur with
  A placenta praevia
  B retention of a dead fetus
  C abruptio placenta
  D amniotic fluid embolus
  E hypovalaemic shock

292 Impacted shoulders
  A are more common in diabetic pregnancies
  B should be delivered with a large episiotomy
  C should be delivered by decapitation
  D should be delivered by Lovset's manoeuvre
  E should be managed in the left lateral position

293 Symptoms of impending eclampsia include
  A loin pain
  B epigastic pain
  C severe headache
  D tinnitus
  E visual disturbances

294 ABO incompatability
  A characteristically affects the primigravid patient
  B occurs most commonly when the mother is group A
  C is usually diagnosed in the antenatal period
  D is associated with a strongly positive Coomb's test
  E may require an exchange transfusion

291 A False
B True
C True
D True
E False

Coagulation defects in pregnancy particularly hypofibrinogenaemia and inappropriate fibrinolysis occurs following release of thromboplastins into the circulation. This occurs following placental abruption, retention of a dead fetus and amniotic fluid embolus. The most common cause is abruptio placentae and it should always be suspected as a cause of excess bleeding either before delivery or as a post-partum haemorrhage.

292 A True
B True
C False
D False
E True

Impacted shoulders or shoulder dystocia constitute a frightening emergency which should be managed promptly as the baby may die or be left with a severe Erb's palsy. The patient should be in the left lateral or in the lithotomy position and a large episiotomy performed. If delivery is not achieved with gentle traction or suprapubic pressure, rotation of the posterior arm through half a circle will solve the problem. Very rarely cleidotomy may be necessary but no other destructive operation is indicated.

293 A False
B True
C True
D False
E True

Eclampsia remains an important cause of maternal and perinatal death particularly in the Third World. Such convulsions are not always preceded by hypertension and proteinuria. Severe headache and visual disturbances are often the first symptoms. Epigastric pain is a feature and a serious sign being the result of subcapsular liver haemorrhages.

294 A True
B False
C False
D False
E True

ABO incompatability usually occurs when the mother is group O and the baby group A. Unlike rhesus disease the first pregnancy may be affected as fetal haemolysis is due to 'natural' antibodies, and not to antibodies induced by iso-immunization. The condition is usually manifest in the first and second day of life and, although not often serious, may require exchange transfusion. The Coomb's test is negative or only weakly positive.

295 The following are known to be harmful to the developing fetus
- **A** smoking
- **B** coitus
- **C** exercise
- **D** swimming
- **E** marihuana

296 Pica
- **A** is an aversion to particular foods in pregnancy
- **B** is rare in developing countries
- **C** is essential to normal fetal growth
- **D** may be diagnosed on abdominal X-ray
- **E** is usually harmless to the fetus and mother

297 In a patient with prolonged pregnancy
- **A** the pregnancy has reached 42 weeks or beyond
- **B** the pregnancy should be monitored by an oxytocin test
- **C** the cervix is characteristically effaced and dilated
- **D** the incidence of meconium staining of the liquor is increased
- **E** labour must be induced

295 A True
    B False
    C False
    D False
    E False

Exercise of any kind is probably beneficial during pregnancy so long as it is not pursued to excess. Coitus is also perfectly safe except where the pregnancy is unstable. There is now clear evidence that smoking is harmful to the fetus. The babies of mothers who smoke are smaller than for non-smoking mothers and have an increased perinatal mortality rate. The effects of smoking marihuana have not been fully evaluated but there do not seem to be any obvious harmful effects.

296 A False
    B False
    C False
    D True
    E True

Pica is a craving in pregnancy for a particular type of food of substance. Usually the craving is for something edible (raw fruit, vegetables etc) but it may be for clay, earth, ant heaps, etc. The practice is widespread throughout the world and unless practised to the exclusion of other foodstuffs is generally harmless. If the patient has been ingesting earth the radio opaque particles will show up clearly on abdominal X-ray. This is usually seen as an incidental finding.

297 A True
    B False
    C False
    D True
    E False

The management of prolonged pregnancy is controversial. Although perinatal mortality is increased after 42 weeks it is possible to identify the fetus at risk if the patient is monitored carefully with appropriate tests. These consist of kick counts, cardiotocography (non-stress tests) and ultrasonic evaluation of fetal growth to ensure that there is no intra-uterine growth retardation. Routine induction is generally not advocated for 'normal postmaturity' but is reserved for patients with some evidence of fetal compromise.

298 A 40-year-old grand multipara who has been in labour for 20 hr complains of sudden onset of lower abdominal pain with a rapid pulse and low blood pressure. On vaginal examination the presenting part cannot be felt. The most likely diagnosis is
- **A** placenta praevia
- **B** uterine rupture
- **C** amniotic fluid embolism
- **D** supine hypotension
- **E** placental abruption

299 Post-partum haemorrhage is associated with
- **A** uterine atony
- **B** amniotic fluid embolism
- **C** acute hepatitis
- **D** twin pregnancy
- **E** prolonged labour

300 Mental retardation is associated with
- **A** cystic fibrosis
- **B** congenital toxoplasmosis
- **C** XY genotype
- **D** fetal alcohol syndrome
- **E** intra-venticular haemorrhage

301 The fetal alcohol syndrome is characterized by
- **A** fetal growth retardation
- **B** renal abnormalities
- **C** spina bifida
- **D** characteristic facies
- **E** cardiac abnormalities

298 A False
B True
C False
D False
E False

Collapse in labour is likely to be due to bleeding (internal or external) or embolism. Being a grand multipara in prolonged labour there is a strong likelihood of uterine rupture. The presenting part commonly recedes from the vagina possibly passing into the peritoneal cavity.

299 A True
B True
C True
D True
E True

A uterus that has been over-filled by hydramnios, a big baby or multiple pregnancy or which has been slow to contract during labour will also be slow to contract after delivery. Amniotic fluid embolism and acute hepatitis are associated with potentially lethal coagulation defects.

300 A False
B True
C False
D True
E True

Fetal alcohol syndrome and also many maternal infections such as rubella, CMV and toxoplasmosis will cause mental retardation. We believe that the normal male genotype is not particularly a great risk factor. The intra-venticular haemorrhage which occurs with prematurity and respiratory distress syndrome greatly influences the long term prognosis of the infant.

301 A True
B True
C False
D True
E True

Alcohol is probably as great a mutagen as rubella. The fetal alcohol syndrome first reported in 1973 produces small for dates infants with permanent stunting of growth, characteristic facies, microcephaly, mental defect with cardiac and renal abnormalities. It follows excessive drinking of any type of alcohol either as steady drinking or 'binge'-ing. Alcohol intake should be discouraged in pregnancy as firmly as smoking.

302 Recurrent mid-trimester abortions occur with
A   chronic renal disease
B   syphilis
C   bicornuate uterus
D   pre-eclampsia
E   fibroids

303 A patient with severe heart disease in pregnancy
A   is managed by induction of labour at term
B   needs prophylactic antibiotics during pregnancy
C   is at greater risk in the mid-trimester
D   needs an assisted delivery
E   should have a lumbar epidural block

304 Physiological changes associated with mid-trimester pregnancy are
A   an increase in cardiac output
B   a pulse rate decreasing by 10 beats/min
C   an increase in blood pressure
D   a decrease in haemoglobin concentration
E   an increase in glomerular filtration

302 **A** True
B True
C True
D False
E True

The classical example of recurrent mid-trimester abortion is in patients with cervical incompetence which may be idiopathic or following termination of pregnancy or cervical surgery. Uterine malformations and fibroids may produce the same clinical problems by distorting the shape of the uterine cavity. Syphilis produces mid-trimester stillbirth followed by abortion. Chronic renal disease has a recurrent hypertensive factor and may produce the same complications but pre-eclampsia is an acute disease usually of the first pregnancy.

303 **A** False
B False
C False
D True
E True

The increased plasma volume in cardiac output increase the risk to patients with cardiac disease early in pregnancy. This risk is maintained towards term when there is a greater load on the heart in the puerperium together with the added risk of bacterial endocarditis. Spontaneous labour should be awaited. There should be adequate analgesia and an assisted second stage will also help reduce the increased cardiac output associated with pain and the maternal expulsive efforts. Antibiotics (gentamicin and a broad spectrum penicillin) should be reserved for labour and the puerperium.

304 **A** True
B False
C False
D True
E True

The increase in cardiac output in normal pregnancy is a result of an increase in heart rate and of stroke volume. The blood pressure usually decreases a little in the mid-trimester. The GFR increases by about 40% hence the normal values for blood urea and creatinine are less in pregnancy. Although there is an increase in total haemoglobin mass in pregnancy, the plasma volume increases greater hence there is a fall in haemoglobin concentration.

305 The complications of post-maturity are
- A   cephalo-pelvic disproportion
- B   increased perinatal mortality
- C   placental insufficiency
- D   hyaline membrane disease
- E   malpresentation

306 A potential diabetic patient may show the following features
- A   a history of babies weighing more than 4 kg
- B   a family history of diabetes
- C   an abnormal glucose tolerance test in pregnancy
- D   glycosuria on two or more occasions in pregnancy
- E   a past history of hypertension

307 Sudden post-partum shock without excessive visible blood loss is caused by
- A   lacerations of the cervix
- B   rupture of the uterus
- C   amniotic fluid embolus
- D   broad ligament haematoma
- E   inversion of the uterus

308 Reliable signs of fetal distress in labour are
- A   excessive fetal movements
- B   meconium staining of the liquor
- C   late decelerations of the fetal heart
- D   fetal scalp pH less than 7.20
- E   fetal tachycardia

305 A True
    B True
    C True
    D False
    E False

Although most normal pregnancies can safely be allowed to proceed beyond term, the risks of inadequate placental perfusion increase and there is an overall increase in perinatal mortality with postmaturity. Such pregnancies require careful antenatal assessment of fetal health. Cephalo-pelvic disproportion is more common although this is not a major problem. Hyaline membrane disease is a feature of prematurity with inadequate surfactant formation. Malpresentations are also more frequent in prematurity but not in post-term pregnancies.

306 A True
    B True
    C False
    D True
    E False

Answers (A), (B) and (D) are all features of a potential diabetic and indicate that a glucose tolerance test should be performed in pregnancy. If this is abnormal (C) the patient is a gestational diabetic and should be managed accordingly. A past history of hypertension is not relevant.

307 A False
    B True
    C True
    D True
    E True

Shock associated with blood loss from a cervical laceration will always present with obvious bleeding. Rupture of the uterus, broad ligament and paravaginal haematomas are also associated with blood loss but this will often be concealed. Amniotic fluid embolus and inversion of the uterus can cause shock in a post-partum patient with no associated blood loss.

308 A False
    B False
    C True
    D True
    E False

Meconium staining of the liquor is a warning sign but in the absence of fetal heart abnormalities does not indicate a distressed fetus. Late decelerations of the fetal heart rate are often associated with hypoxic fetuses and this is confirmed if the fetal scalp pH is less than 7.20. A fetal tachycardia may not signify a distressed fetus and can be present where there is a maternal pyrexia or dehydration.

309 The pain associated with uterine contractions

   A   can be abolished by blocking spinal segments S2, 3, 4

   B   can be abolished by blocking spinal segments T11, 12

   C   is due to tissue anoxia

   D   increases cardiac output

   E   may be reproduced by dilating the cervix

310 The complications of abruptio placenta include

   A   post-partum haemorrhage

   B   malpresentation

   C   hypofibrinogenaemia

   D   fetal death

   E   polyhydramnios

311 In which of the following conditions is the incidence of prolapsed cord increased:

   A   breech presentation

   B   severe cardiac disease

   C   polyhydramnios

   D   placenta praevia

   E   post-maturity

312 Ante-partum haemorrhage

   A   is bleeding from the genital tract at any time in pregnancy

   B   may be caused by cervical erosion

   C   would normally require admission of the patient

   D   occurs in 15% of all pregnancies

   E   should be managed by immediate delivery

309 A False
    B True
    C False
    D True
    E True

The initial stimulus to pain appreciation is unknown, but the pain fibres from the uterus all pass to the spinal segments T11 and 12. Painful contractions cause a greater increase in cardiac output than when the pain is removed, for example by means of a regional block. Uterine pain is blocked by a lumbar epidural block but not by the pudendal block of S2, 3 and 4.

310 A True
    B False
    C True
    D True
    E False

Severe abruptio placenta will nearly always cause fetal death. Activation of the coagulation and fibrinolytic systems will lead to hypofibrinogenaemia and excessive fibrinolysis: post-partum haemorrhage is common and because of the muscle relaxant and anti-coagulant properties of fibrin degradation products. The combination of hypovolaemia, tissue damage and disseminated intravascular coagulation may lead to acute renal failure.

311 A True
    B False
    C True
    D True
    E False

Any condition which discourages the presenting part from entering the pelvic brim will increase the chance of a prolapsed cord. Hence placenta praevia, polyhydramnios and disproportion are major causes. It is also common in breech presentation if the presentation is a footling or a flexed breech.

312 A False
    B True
    C True
    D False
    E False

Ante-partum haemorrhage occurs in 3% of pregnancies and is defined as bleeding from the genital tract after the twenty-eighth week of pregnancy (before that it is designated an abortion but may be equally dangerous). The three main causes are placenta praevia, abruptio plancenta and local cause such as cervical lesions. Such a patient should be admitted for bed rest and investigation but the timing and the mode of delivery will depend on the cause, gestational age and severity of bleeding.

313 Induction of labour is contra-indicated
A where a previous LSCS has been performed for cephalo-pelvic disproportion
B in severe pregnancy-induced hypertension
C in multiparous patients
D in the presence of fetal growth retardation
E where the lie of the fetus is transverse

314 Chorio amnionitis
A is characteristically accompanied by a pyrexia
B occurs in 25% of all pregnancies
C is an important cause of post-maturity
D occurs in the presence of intact membranes
E is more common in patients of the low income groups

315 A partogram is used to
A facilitate recognition of dysfunctional labour
B record the events of pregnancy
C record the events of labour
D establish the gestational age of a fetus
E estimate the date of delivery

316 The following are chromosomal disorders
A Edwards' syndrome
B haemophilia
C Turner's syndrome
D Klinefelter's syndrome
E muscular dystrophy

313 A True
B False
C False
D False
E True

Induction of labour commits obstetricians to delivery in 24 hr and must not be performed for trivial medical or social reasons. Induction should not be undertaken in a patient where a previous Caesarean section has been performed for a recurrent cause or where the lie of the fetus is other than longitudinal.

314 A False
B False
C False
D True
E True

Chorio amnionitis is a common cause of pre-term labour, particularly in patients of lower socioeconomic groups. It certainly occurs in the presence of intact membranes and often there is no accompanying temperature. Venereal infections are a common aetiological factor which lead to a mixed growth infection in the amniotic fluid and infection of the fetus with intra-uterine pneumonia or septicaemia.

315 A True
B False
C True
D False
E False

A graphic labour record or partogram gives a graphic display of all events in labour against a time scale. Its central feature is the cervicograph indicating progress of labour by progressive dilatation of the cervix and by progressive descent of the head. It is educational, clarifying the understanding of labour and by the use of an action line aids the recognition and the treatment of dysfunctional labour.

316 A True
B False
C True
D True
E False

Edwards' syndrome is trisomy 18 and is characterized by microcephaly, heart disease and abnormal feet. Other important trisomies are Down's syndrome trisomy 21 and Patav's syndrome trisomy 13. Turner's syndrome is XO, Klinefelter's syndrome XXY and although haemophilia and muscular dystrophy are sex-linked, they do not have an abnormal chromosomal complement.

317 The following drugs are known to adversely effect the fetus when prescribed during pregnancy
- **A**   tetracycline
- **B**   stilboestrol
- **C**   coumarin anti-coagulants
- **D**   diazepam
- **E**   alcohol

318 Fetoscopy can be used to diagnose
- **A**   sickle cell disease
- **B**   growth retardation
- **C**   hare lip
- **D**   neural tube defects
- **E**   congenital nephrotic syndrome

319 Sickle cell disease in pregnancy is associated with
- **A**   bone infarction
- **B**   urinary infections
- **C**   placental insufficiency
- **D**   hypertension
- **E**   decreased risk of crisis in pregnancy

320 Fetal ascites is caused by
- **A**   fetal congenital heart disease
- **B**   alpha thalassaemia
- **C**   ABO incompatability
- **D**   toxoplasmosis
- **E**   rhesus incompatability

317 A True
B True
C True
D True
E True

Tetracycline causes discoloration and weakening of the teeth, stilboestrol may produce vaginal adenosis or clear cell carcinoma 20 years after intra-uterine exposure. Coumarin may produce placental or fetal haemorrhage. Diazepam causes hypotonia and hypothermia and alcohol causes the fetal alcohol syndrome. It is best to attempt to avoid all but life-saving drugs during pregnancy, particularly during the first trimester.

318 A True
B False
C True·
D True
E False

The examination of the fetus by a small needlescope can diagnose major abnormalities such as spina bifida and hare lip. It is also possible to take a sample of the fetal blood to diagnose sickle cell disease, haemophilia or beta thalassaemia. In skilled hands it is a safe procedure with only a 1% incidence of premature labour or abortion.

319 A True
B True
C False
D False
E False

Sickle cell disease has a greatly increased maternal and perinatal mortality, and there is an increased risk of crisis in pregnancy. This latter problem can be prevented by exchange or 'top up' blood transfusions of normal blood thus decreasing the percentage of haemoglobin S or haemoglobin C. Hypertension is not a feature of sickle cell disease, nor is placental insufficiency.

320 A True
B True
C False
D False
E True

There are several causes of fetal ascites which can now be recognized at an early stage by ultrasonography. Rhesus incompatability is the commonest cause in the U.K. and alpha thalassaemia, which is incompatible with life is most common in Asia and in Mediterranean countries.

321 Fetoscopy is used for diagnosis of
   A   haemophilia
   B   thalassaemia major
   C   hydrocephalus
   D   cleft palate
   E   congenital heart disease

322 An occipito-posterior position in labour
   A   characteristically delivers spontaneously face to pubis
   B   is often deflexed
   C   undergoes short rotation to occipito-anterior
   D   presents the occipito-frontal diameter
   E   is associated with an increased incidence of congenital ab-
          normalities

323 The following should be used in the management of multiple pregnancy:
   A   elective Shirodkar suture
   B   admission at 30 weeks for bed rest
   C   serial urinary oestriols
   D   dietary supplements of iron and folic acid
   E   normal antenatal care

324 Useful placental function tests are:
   A   haemoglobin A1
   B   HPL
   C   urinary oestriols
   D   Papp-A
   E   HCG

321 A True   The potential of fetoscopy for diagnosis is increas-
    B True   ing as one is able to recognize several chromosomal
    C False abnormalities and metabolic disorders as well as all
    D True   of the haemoglobinopathies. It also has a thera-
    E False peutic use with intra-uterine transfusion for rhesus
             disease and bladder catherization for the treatment
             of outflow obstruction.

322 A True   An occipito-posterior position in labour usually
    B True   undergoes long rotation to an occipito-anterior
    C False position but it may deliver face to pubis. The head
    D True   is often deflexed presenting the occipito-frontal dia-
    E False meter and abnormal uterine action may occur with
             dysfunctional labour. Delivery may be with a
             vacuum extractor, forceps delivery face to pubis or
             after rotation with Kjelland's forceps to an occipito-
             anterior position.

323 A False Most obstetric complications (except post-
    B False maturity) are more likely with multiple pregnancy.
    C False The normal routine antenatal care will detect most
    D True   of these. Although prematurity is common,
    E True   Shirodkar suture does not help and routine admis-
             sion at 30 weeks for bed rest does not reduce its
             frequency. Placental insufficiency and fetal growth
             retardation are more common than in singleton
             pregnancies but urinary oestriols are inappropriate
             for this, serial ultrasound being preferred.

324 A False A difficult question because fashions in placental
    B False function tests have changed so quickly. HPL and
    C False 24-hr urinary oestriol have been so disappointing
    D False that they are scarcely used now. Haemoglobin A1 is
    E False used to assess efficiency of diabetic control and the
             placental protein Papp-A although an interesting
             substance seems to be without a clinical use. Per-
             haps the best indirect placental function tests are
             fetal movements and ultrasonic assessment of fetal
             growth.

325 Placenta praevia
A   causes painless vaginal bleeding
B   is managed by Caesarean section if Grade I or II
C   is associated with breech presentation
D   predisposes to post-partum haemorrhage
E   presents with a woody hard uterus on palpation

326 Abruptio placentae
A   usually causes a low blood pressure
B   frequently needs central venous pressure monitoring
C   is a non-recurrent cause of APH
D   causes a Couvelaire uterus
E   causes acute cortical necrosis

327 A patient at 28 weeks' gestation is found to have an intramural fibroid in which red degeneration is occurring. Which of the following forms of management would be appropriate:
A   bed rest and antibiotic therapy
B   bed rest and analgesics
C   exploratory laparotomy with myomectomy
D   Caesarean hysterectomy
E   Interstitial injection with 1% xylocaine

328 Grand multigravidae are liable to
A   malpresentation
B   pre-eclampsia
C   placenta praevia
D   post-partum haemorrhage
E   rupture of uterus

325 A True
    B False
    C True
    D True
    E False

Placenta praevia usually presents with recurrent painless bleeding which may be heavy. The management is conservative until approximately 38 weeks, unless heavy bleeding necessitates urgent delivery in order to save the mother's life. It is associated with prematurity and hence breech presentation. The lower segment site of the placenta does not retract well in the third stage and therefore post-partum haemorrhage is more common.

326 A False
    B True
    C False
    D True
    E True

The bleeding of an abruption may be severe although this blood loss may be revealed or completely concealed. Nevertheless, blood pressure is usually normal or even high due to peripheral vaso constriction. A central venous pressure line is usually required in order to monitor adequate fluid and blood replacement and prevent circulatory collapse with acute tubular or cortical necrosis.

327 A False
    B True
    C False
    D False
    E False

Red degeneration (necrobiosis) is venous infarction of the rapidly growing fibroid during pregnancy. Treatment is conservative with bed rest and analgesia and any form of surgery is strongly contraindicated. The danger is that the condition is so similar to an acute appendicitis with a leukocytosis pyrexia and raised ESR that a laparotomy may be performed unwisely.

328 A True
    B False
    C False
    D True
    E True

Malpresentations and larger babies are more common in grand multiparous patients hence the risk of uterine rupture increases. Although uterine contractions during labour are strong and indeed are dangerously strong when obstruction of labour occurs, retraction in the third stage is less good and post-partum haemorrhage is more common. Preeclampsia tends to occur in primigravid women but chronic hypertensive disease is commoner in the older and multigravid women.

329 The following statements concerning breech presentation are true:

A   there is an association with hydrocephaly
B   it is associated with uterine abnormality
C   incidence is 5–10%
D   an extended breech characteristically has a greater risk of cord prolapse
E   an abdominal X-ray or ultrasound scan should always be done

330 The following drugs are effective and safe:

A   pethidine in the first stage of labour
B   nikethamide for infant resuscitation
C   marcaine in patients with cardiac disease
D   salbutamol in false labour
E   prophylactic antibiotics with premature membranes rupture

331 The following signs suggest that cephalopelvic disproportion is present in labour:

A   increasing fetal skull moulding
B   fetal head two-fifths above the pelvic brim
C   fetal heart acceleration during contractions
D   dysfunctional labour
E   meconium-staining of the liquor

329 **A** True
B True
C False
D False
E False

In most populations the incidence of breech presentation is 3–5% being more common with prematurity. Abnormalities in the uterine cavity predispose to malpresentation as does fetal abnormality in the form of hydrocephalis or weak or paralysed feet which prevent spontaneous version to cephalic presentation. Abnormality should be excluded by X-ray or ultrasound examination. A footling or a frank breech predisposes to cord presentation or prolapse.

330 **A** False
B False
C True
D False
E False

If pethidine is given late in the first stage of labour there is a risk of respiratory depression in the neonate. This should be treated with intubation and ventilation. Nikethamide and other stimulants have no place in the management of this problem. Beta-sympathomimetic drugs such as salbutamol can be used in pre-term labour but are unnecessary in false labour. There is a risk of intra-uterine and fetal infection with premature membrane rupture but prophylactic antibiotics only create neonatal problems of bacterial resistance.

331 **A** True
B False
C False
D True
E False

Cephalopelvic disproportion may be suspected in patients with a clinically or radiologically small pelvis, in patients of small stature with a high-head at term, but the only way to diagnose cephalopelvic disproportion is by a trial of labour. Dysfunctional labour (i.e. slow labour), in spite of oxytocin stimulation and the finding of excessive skull moulding strongly suggests the diagnosis.

332 The following malpresentations occurring in a near term fetus can be delivered safely by the vaginal route

A breech presentation
B brow presentation
C mento posterior face presentation
D shoulder presentation
E cord presentation

333 Meconium-staining of the amniotic fluid in labour

A is a poor indicator of fetal distress
B increases the risk of intra-amniotic infection
C indicates that careful fetal monitoring should be instituted
D may lead to respiratory difficulties in the neonate
E rarely occurs before 32 weeks' gestation

334 Neville Barnes' or Simpson's forceps delivery at full dilatation may be performed for the following indications:

A an occipito-posterior position of the head
B a brow presentation
C cardiac disease in the mother
D poor maternal effort
E deep transverse arrest

332 A True
B False
C False
D False
E False

Breech presentations can be delivered vaginally provided careful ante-partum assessments of pelvic capacity and the fetal size have been made. A brow presentation cannot be delivered but a mento-anterior face presenting the submento-bregmatic diameter can usually be delivered vaginally. A shoulder presentation needs a Caesarean section and a cord presentation occurs with the membranes intact and urgent delivery is required before a cord prolapse occurs.

333 A True
B False
C True
D True
E True

Meconium-staining of the liquor is the least valuable sign of fetal distress and, if significant, co-exists with more dramatic signs such as fetal growth retardation, oligohydramnios and fetal heart abnormalities. It is uncommon in a premature fetus and is very rare before 32 weeks. There is a strong association with post-maturity and a danger of meconium aspiration and pneumonitis particularly when the fetus shows other signs of hypoxia in utero.

334 A True
B False
C True
D True
E False

An occipito-posterior position and poor maternal effort due to tiredness or an epidural block will cause delay in the second stage and are all indications for mid-cavity forceps delivery. It would be safe to deliver an occipito-posterior position face to pubis if the head is low in the pelvis. Forceps should be used in cardiac disease in order to prevent excessive maternal effort. A deep transverse arrest should be rotated by Kjelland's forceps or by hand before delivery. A brow presentation should be delivered by Caesarean section.

335 Characteristics of Kjelland's forceps are
  A the English lock
  B no pelvic curve
  C the ability to correct asynclitism
  D use in breech delivery
  E use for the difficult mid-cavity delivery

336 Complications of external cephalic version include
  A rhesus isoimmunization
  B breech presentation
  C premature labour
  D fetal distress
  E cord rupture

337 Pregnancy at 20 weeks' gestation can be positively confirmed by
  A ultrasound
  B pregnancy test on the urine
  C palpition of the fetal parts
  D symptoms of nausea and vomiting
  E X-ray

335 A False
B True
C True
D False
E False

Kjelland's forceps are used for rotation and traction, thus they have a cephalic curve but no pelvic curve. There is a sliding lock which enables correction of asynclitism (lateral flexion). They are also used to rotate from an occipito-posterior position or a deep transverse arrest to an occipito-anterior position before traction and delivery. They should not, nor should any other forceps, be used for difficult mid-cavity deliveries.

336 A True
B False
C True
D True
E False

External cephalic version is used to convert a breech presentation to cephalic. It has a small place in practice but should be carried out with extreme gentleness. Complications include a feto maternal haemorrhage which may immunize if the mother is rhesus negative and the baby rhesus positive. Premature labour may occur because of placental separation or premature membranes rupture. These may cause fetal distress; as may cord prolapse or a true knot in the cord.

337 A True
B False
C False
D False
E True

Both abdominal X-ray and ultrasound will detect a fetus at 20 weeks' gestation but ultrasound is by far the more preferable procedure. An X-ray probably carries a very small risk of causing leukaemia in the offspring later in life. A standard urinary pregnancy test may be negative at this time. It is usually too early to hear the fetal heart by auscultation but it would be easily picked up by ultrasound. Fetal parts are not palpable until week 26. Nausea and vomiting may be due to other causes.

338 **Syphilis in pregnancy**
  A   causes mid-trimester intra-uterine death
  B   is usually diagnosed by serology
  C   is treated with 2 days of procaine penicillin
  D   should be treated until serological tests become negative
  E   causes hypertension

339 **A 'large for dates' uterus may be due to**
  A   cephalo-pelvic disproportion
  B   multiple pregnancy
  C   spina bifida
  D   hydatidiform mole
  E   error in dates

340 **Cephalhaematoma**
  A   is oedema occurring over the presenting part of the head
  B   disappears within a few hours of birth
  C   is often unilateral
  D   may follow a normal delivery
  E   should be aspirated

341 **The following drugs can be used for prophylaxis against malaria in pregnancy**
  A   pyrimethamine
  B   quinine
  C   metronidiazole
  D   chloroquine
  E   danazol

338 A True
    B True
    C False
    D False
    E False

Syphilis is still a very important cause of perinatal mortality in many developing countries, accounting for up to 10% of perinatal deaths in some places. A screening test such as the VDRL test is usually used as a routine with more specific tests such as the *Troponema pallidum* immobilization test (TPI) or fluorescent antibody absorption test (FTA) for confirmation. The treatment should be with long-acting penicillin (benzathine penicillin) weekly for 3 weeks or with a full course of 14 days crystalline penicillin. The serological tests will often remain positive for a long time after treatment.

339 A False
    B True
    C True
    D True
    E True

The most common cause of a 'large for dates' uterus is wrong dates. It may also result from multiple pregnancy, hydatidiform mole, macrosomia (for example, in diabetic pregnancies), fibroids and any cause of polyhydramnios (spina bifida). Ultrasonic scanning will clarify virtually all these causes.

340 A False
    B False
    C True
    D True
    E False

Cephalhaematoma is a fluctant swelling due to extravasation of blood under the periosteum. Because of the periosteal attachment it may be unilateral. It may present up to 36 hr after birth and is treated conservatively. Aspiration should be avoided because of the risk of infection. It is important to distinguish cephalhaematoma from caput succedaneum, which presents at birth and usually disappears in the first 12 hr.

341 A True
    B False
    C False
    D True
    E False

The serious effects that malaria has on the outcome of pregnancy make the use of prophylactics mandatory in areas where the disease is common. Quinine has been superseded by more effective and safer synthetic compounds. Chloroquine and primethamine are excellent suppressants and can be taken weekly.

342 An episiotomy

    A   should nearly always be performed in primigravid deliveries

    B   does not need a local anaesthetic

    C   is indicated in post-maturity

    D   may be medial or postero lateral

    E   should be performed in breech deliveries

343 The degree of rhesus isoimmunization can be detected in utero by

    A   maternal antibody levels

    B   amniotic fluid bilirubin levels

    C   amniotic fluid oestriol levels

    D   ultrasound scanning

    E   maternal serum alpha-fetoprotein levels

344 Cervical lacerations which are bleeding heavily after delivery

    A   occur after normal delivery

    B   should be sutured immediately

    C   should be packed

    D   may extend into the body of the uterus

    E   are best identified by digital examination

345 Ergometrine

    A   given intravenously causes the uterus to contract in 45 sec

    B   causes contraction of both upper and lower uterine segments

    C   given intramuscularly acts in 7 min

    D   given intravenously often causes a drop in blood pressure

    E   given by intravenous drip in the first stage of labour improves the efficiency of uterine action

342 A False
    B False
    C False
    D True
    E True

The episiotomy is a valuable obstetric procedure which should be performed only when there is an appropriate indication. The posterior-lateral type is the more frequently used. The medial site is less painful but runs a great risk of extending to a third degree tear. The perineum should always be infused with local anaesthetic and the indications include mid-cavity forceps, pre-term labour and breech delivery.

343 A False
    B True
    C False
    D True
    E False

Raised anti-D antibody levels in the maternal serum do not confirm that the fetus in utero is affected as the fetus in the current pregnancy may be rhesus negative. The most reliable method is measurement of amniotic fluid bilirubin levels by spectrophotometry at optical density 450 mμ. Rising levels usually indicate an affected fetus. Ultrasound scanning can identify hydrops fetalis.

344 A True
    B True
    C False
    D True
    E False

Cervical lacerations may follow a normal delivery although they are more common after an operative vaginal delivery. They may extend to the lower segment or the body of the uterus involving the uterine vessels. They are identified by a careful speculum examination with proper assistance and a good light. They should be sutured as soon as possible and packing has no place in the management of this serious complication.

345 A True
    B True
    C True
    D False
    E False

Ergometrine is given alone or in combination with syntocinon as syntometrine at the birth of the anterior shoulder or at the crowning of the head. It causes contraction of the uterine muscle but cannot be used in the first stage of labour as the contraction is persistent and hypertonia and fetal distress or death could result. Care must be taken with intravenous ergometrine in hypertensive patients as it causes an increase in the blood pressure in the immediate puerperum.

346 **Maternal pyrexia in the puerperium may be due to**
  A   engorged breasts
  B   deep vein thrombosis
  C   involution of the uterus
  D   post-partum depression
  E   malaria

347 **The following drugs are absolutely contra-indicated in the breast-feeding mother**
  A   methotrexate
  B   tetracycline
  C   ampicillin
  D   diazepam
  E   phenobarbitone

348 **At the sixth week post-natal examination the patient should have the following features checked:**
  A   subinvolution
  B   retroversion
  C   cervical erosion
  D   birth control
  E   haemoglobin level

349 **At 6 weeks a baby should**
  A   follow with eyes
  B   still have a Moro reflex
  C   have the hips tested
  D   have no palpable anterior fontanelle
  E   smile

346 A True
B True
C False
D False
E True

Engorged breasts can cause a rise in temperature without other evidence of infection ('milk fever'). Deep vein thrombosis is particularly liable to occur in the puerperium but is rare in developing countries. Malaria, however, is commonly seen in the puerperium as often the attack of malaria has precipitated labour. Involution of the uterus and post-partum depression do not cause a rise in maternal temperature.

347 A True
B False
C False
D False
E False

All cytotoxic agents will affect the baby and should not be used in breast-feeding women. In general all medication should be avoided where possible but the concentration of the other drugs listed above do not cross to the baby in levels high enough for them to be absolutely contra-indicated when they are necessary.

348 A False
B False
C False
D True
E True

Six weeks represent the end of the puerperium and the time when breast feeding should be established and all the changes of pregnancy have returned to normal. Episiotomy or Caesarean section scars should be examined and it is worth while checking the haemoglobin in preparation for the hard work ahead for the mother. Traditionally obstetricians used to check for subinvolution, retroversion and erosions, but as these findings should not be treated it is a worthless exercise. The most important functions of the post-natal clinic is to give advice on birth control and to admire the baby.

349 A True
B True
C True
D False
E True

The sixth week visit to the baby clinic should consist of a general examination and particularly the weight, head circumference, hips and the heart, as murmurs of a VSD may be present which were absent at birth. The baby should turn to sound, fix and follow with eyes, smile and still have the Moro reflex which will disappear at about 16 weeks. The closure of the anterior fontanelle is variable between 4 months and 20 months with 18 months as the usually stated time.

350 In the normal puerperium
- **A** the uterine fundus is no longer palpable abdominally after 7 days
- **B** a diuresis occurs in the first 24 hr
- **C** retention of urine occurs
- **D** ovulation is usually re-established
- **E** red lochia continues for up to 6 weeks

351 Premature rupture of the membranes
- **A** should be treated with betamethazone
- **B** means rupture of the membranes before contractions begin
- **C** should be diagnosed by a digital vaginal examination
- **D** predisposes to intra-uterine pneumonia
- **E** means rupture of the membranes before term

352 Smoking in pregnancy is associated with:
- **A** late booking
- **B** low incidence of breast feeding
- **C** low birth weight
- **D** lower I.Q. of child
- **E** lower socio-economic group of mother

350 A False
B True
C True
D False
E False

The puerperium is a time when physiological changes of pregnancy return to normal and breast feeding is established. The duration is 6 weeks. The uterus is usually not palpable abdominally by 10–14 days and the passage of red lochia is usually complete by day 14. Although a diuresis occurs early in the puerperium, retention of urine occurs as a result of trauma at delivery and catheterization may be necessary. Ovulation rarely occurs before 6 weeks even if the patient does not breast feed.

351 A False
B True
C False
D True
E False

Premature rupture of the membranes can occur at any period of gestation. It is defined as spontaneous rupture of the membranes before contractions begin. Perhaps the most important act is to prevent infection (chorio amnionitis, fetal pneumonia and septicaemia) by not performing a digital vaginal examination. The condition is usually treated conservatively up to week 34 of pregnancy but contractions are induced by oxytocin after that gestation.

352 A True
B True
C True
D True
E True

There is no doubt that there is a considerable pharmacological element (either due to increased carboxy-haemoglobin or vasospasm with nicotine) which causes fetal growth retardation and a higher perinatal mortality. However, the associated social factors are important and include low socio-economic group, unemployment, late booking, poor attendance at the antenatal clinic, being unsure of dates, etc. with a disinclination to breast feed completing the sad picture.

353 Amniotic fluid embolus:
A   usually occurs in the puerperium
B   is usually fatal
C   is associated with hypofibrogenaemia
D   is associated with the use of oxytoxics
E   is more common in primigravid patients

354 The following increase the risk of post-partum haemorrhage
A   syntometrine in the third stage of labour
B   multiple pregnancy
C   operative vaginal delivery
D   previous post-partum haemorrhage
E   polyhydramnios

355 Primary post-partum haemorrhage
A   occurs within 24 hr of delivery
B   is associated with retained blood clot
C   is more common after acceleration of labour
D   is responsible for more maternal deaths than ante-partum haemorrhage
E   is diagnosed when blood loss exceeds 200 ml

356 The following factors increase the risk of genital tract infection in the puerperium
A   failure to wear a mask at delivery
B   retained piece of placental tissue
C   fetal blood sampling
D   prolonged labour
E   meconium-staining of the liquor

353 A False
B True
C True
D True
E False

Amniotic fluid embolus is a sudden devastating and usually fatal complication which characteristically occurs in the first stage of labour particularly in the presence of strong contractions in a multigravida or following augmentation with oxytocin. Death may be sudden or life may be threatened by complicating haemorrhage as amniotic fluid thromboplastin enters the circulation and removes fibrinogen.

354 A False
B True
C True
D True
E True

Post-partum haemorrhage tends to be recurrent as the same risk factors are operative. Multiple pregnancy and polyhydramnios cause overdistension. Multiparity and placental abruption also predispose to the atonic type of PPH. Operative vaginal delivery increases the chance of traumatic haemorrhage from vaginal, cervical or lower segment tears. The use of syntometrine will reduce the risk of post-partum haemorrhage although the incidence of retained placenta may be increased.

355 A True
B True
C False
D True
E False

Primary post-partum haemorrhage is usually defined as bleeding from the birth canal in excess of 500 ml occurring within 24 hr of delivery. The incidence can be reduced by the use of oxytocic drugs in the active management of the third stage of labour. Retained products of conception or blood clot constitute one of the four major causes of post-partum haemorrhage. The others are trauma, uterine atony and coagulation defects.

356 A False
B True
C False
D True
E True

Examinations in labour should be performed with sterile precautions but the presence of a mask is not necessary and is also intimidating to the mother. Prolonged labour will increase the risk of infection, particularly if many vaginal examinations are performed. Meconium is a good culture medium and removes the normal bacteriocidal properties of amniotic fluid.

202

357 **Bacteriuria in pregnancy**
A   occurs in 5–10% of pregnant women
B   predisposes to acute pyelonephritis
C   is more common in primigravid patients
D   should be treated with antibiotics
E   is normally associated with proteinuria

358 **A primigravida is admitted at 40 weeks' gestation with a pulsatile prolapsed umbilical cord. The cervix is 8 cm dilated, the head not engaged. Treatment should be:**
A   await spontaneous delivery
B   vacuum extraction
C   Duhurssen's incision and forceps delivery
D   internal podalic version and breech extraction
E   Caesarean section

CASE HISTORY

A 30-year-old primigravida is admitted to the labour ward complaining of painless vaginal bleeding. She is at 39 weeks of gestation. Uterine size is consistent with this, the presentation is cephalic, the head five-fifths palpable and the uterus soft. The pulse rate is 100 beats/min, the blood pressure 110/70 mmHg and the bleeding is slight but persistent. The fetal heart rate is normal.

359 **The following steps are important:**
A   check blood urea level
B   request blood to be cross-matched
C   perform a digital vaginal examination
D   request ultrasound scan
E   commence intravenous infusion

The bleeding is persistent and painful uterine contractions commence.

360 **The following management is appropriate:**
A   induction of labour by artificial rupture of membranes
B   induction of labour by oxytocin infusion
C   intravenous salbutamol
D   intra-muscular steroids
E   examination in the operating theatre

357 **A** True   Bacteria can be cultured from the urine in 5–10%
     B True   of pregnant women. Significant bacteriuria
     C False   (> 100,000 organisms/ml) should be treated usually
     D True   with ampicillin as clinical acute pyelonephritis may
     E False   occur in 25% of these patients. There is also an
                      increased incidence of hypertension, fetal growth
                      retardation and perinatal loss. Antibiotic therapy is
                      effective in preventing the acute infection but does
                      little to help, the other complications which are
                      related to the underlying chronic renal disease.

358 **A** False   In umbilical cord prolapse the best fetal salvage is
     B False   obtained by Caesarean section. In the multiparous
     C False   patient with the cervix fully dilated, instrumental
     D False   delivery may be indicated. If the fetus is already
     E True   dead, vaginal delivery should be awaited and the
                      uterus therefore left intact.

CASE HISTORY

359 **A** False   Any patient who is bleeding must have blood taken
     B True   for grouping and cross-matching, and an intra-
     C False   venous infusion commenced. Checking blood urea
     D False   level is irrelevant and ultrasound scan is not
     E True   appropriate as bleeding is active and the findings
                      will not alter management at this stage of gestation.

360 **A** False   The baby is mature, the most important element of
     B False   differentiation diagnosis is placenta praevia and
     C False   delivery is appropriate. This must be preceded by
     D False   examination in the operating theatre (sometimes
     E True   under anaesthesia) to determine the mode of
                      delivery.

Examination in theatre reveals the placenta to be covering the os and felt in the anterior vaginal fornix. The bleeding is slight.

361 The following proceedures are appropriate:
A   hind water rupture
B   lower segment Caesarean section
C   classical Caesarean section
D   vaginal packing and await delivery
E   acceleration of labour

CASE HISTORY

A 26-year-old primigravid patient presents in the labour ward in labour. Her LMP is 17.3.82; her periods have been regular and she has not taken oral contraceptives. She is 150 cm tall. On examination the fetus is in longitudinal lie, cephalic presentation, the head four-fifths palpable and the fetal heart is heard. Vaginal examination reveals the cervix to be effaced and 4 cm dilated.

362 The following statements are correct:
A   her EDD is 12.12.82
B   the position of the back of the fetus is of great importance
C   the head is not engaged
D   a persistent slight blood loss pv is to be expected
E   artificial rupture of the membranes should be performed

When the membranes of the above patient are ruptured the amniotic fluid is found to be lightly meconium-stained.

363 The following procedures should be undertaken:
A   the patient should count fetal movements
B   Caesarean section
C   fetal blood sampling
D   continuous fetal heart rate monitoring
E   setting up an oxytocin drip

361 A False
B True
C False
D False
E False

The only acceptable treatment for major placenta praevia is Caesarean section. Except under particular circumstances this should be performed through the lower segment.

CASE HISTORY

362 A False
B False
C True
D False
E True

Present-day convention is to describe the station of the fetal head by how much of the head is palpable per abdomen (fifths). When less than half is palpable it is engaged. A head is engaged or not engaged depending on whether the widest diameter has passed through the pelvic brim. It is never one-fifth engaged etc. The position of the fetal back is only of importance when determining where to listen for the fetal heart sounds. A persistent blood loss is abnormal. The management of established labour includes rupturing the fetal membranes during vaginal examination to inspect the amniotic fluid and possibly apply a fetal scalp electrode.

363 A False
B False
C False
D True
E False

Meconium staining of the amniotic fluid is associated with fetal distress in some cases. It is an indication to monitor the fetus: in labour this is done by continuous electronic fetal heart rate monitoring. If that is abnormal, fetal blood sample or immediate delivery may be necessary. Oxytocin should not be given unless labour becomes abnormal.

The continuous fetal heart rate tracing is normal but at the next vaginal examination 4 hr later the cervix is only 5 cm dilated.

364 The following procedures should be undertaken:
  A   a Caesarean section
  B   clinical pelvimetry
  C   radiological pelvimetry
  D   determination of the position of the occiput
  E   setting up an oxytocin drip

Over the next 4 hr the oxytocin drip rate is escalated to 20 milliunits/ min and the uterus is observed to be contracting regularly and frequently. At the next review the fetal head remains three-fifths palpable per abdomen. Vaginal examination reveals the cervix to be 6 cm dilated. There is marked degree of caput formation and moulding. It is left occipito-transverse position. The presenting part is at the level of the ischial spines.

365 The following are true:
  A   the diagnosis is incoordinate uterine action
  B   vacuum delivery (ventouse) is appropriate
  C   prostaglandins are appropriate treatment
  D   the diagnosis is cephalopelvic disproportion
  E   Caesarean section is appropriate

364 A False
B True
C False
D True
E True

Failure of the cervix to dilate at 1 cm/hr is abnormal labour progress. The possibility of inefficient uterine action, cephalopelvic disproportion or occipito-posterior position should be considered. The patient is short (150 cm) and clinical pelvic assessment should be performed to determine the gross dimension of the birth canal. Radiological pelvimetry will not contribute useful extra information. Cephalopelvic disproportion will not be confirmed until a well-documented trial of labour has failed to deliver the baby. This involves the use of an oxytocin drip as does the treatment of occipito-posterior position and inefficient uterine action.

365 A False
B False
C False
D True
E True

At this stage the inefficient uterine action has been corrected and the position of the occiput is not posterior. The presence of a marked amount of moulding with an unengaged head is diagnostic of cephalopelvic disproportion. Caesarean section is the correct management.